THE HEART
IN LING SHU CHAPTER 8

AcuMedic CENTRE
101-105 CAMDEN HIGH STREET
LONDON NW1 7JN
Tel: 020 7388-6704/5783
info@acumedic.com www.acumedic.com

MONKEY PRESS

Monkey Press is named after the Monkey King in The Journey to the West, the 16th century novel by Wu Chengen. Monkey blends skill, initiative and wisdom with the spirit of freedom, irreverence and a touch of mischief.

CHINESE MEDICINE FROM THE CLASSICS

Also in this series:

The Secret Treatise of the Spiritual Orchid
The Lung
The Kidneys
The Spleen and Stomach
Heart Master, Triple Heater
The Liver
The Way of Heaven: Suwen chapters 1 and 2
Essence, Spirit, Blood and Qi
The Seven Emotions
The Eight Extraordinary Meridians
The Extraordinary Fu

CHINESE MEDICINE FROM THE CLASSICS

Claude Larre and Elisabeth Rochat de la Vallée

THE HEART
in Ling shu chapter 8

A Monkey Press Publication

Published by
MONKEY PRESS
www.monkeypress.net
monkey.press@virgin.net

CHINESE MEDICINE FROM THE CLASSICS:
THE HEART in Ling shu chapter 8
Claude Larre and Elisabeth Rochat de la Vallée
First edition 1991

© Monkey Press 2004

All rights reserved. No part of this book may be reproduced in any form without written permission from the publisher.

ISBN 1 872468 04 7

Transcribed from a seminar organised by Peter Firebrace

Transcribed by Carline Root
Text Editors: Caroline Root and Sandra Hill
Production and Design: Sandra Hill
Calligraphy: Qu Lei Lei
Printed by RapSpiderweb

CONTENTS

Foreword	VI
Introduction	1
The Emperor's Question	18
The Minister's Reply	34
Summary	91
Appendix 1	105
Appendix 2	111
Text and Translation	121

FOREWORD

The Su wen and Ling shu, the two parts of the Huangdi Neijing, are rightly considered foundation texts of Chinese medicine. The framework of man, *ren*, between heaven and earth, *tian di*, is ever-present. The alternating flux of *yin yang*, the turning of the four seasons, *si shi*, the dynamic interplay of the five phases, *wu xing*, this is the field of medicine, the field of the *zangfu*, the organs, whose interrelationships were studied in Su wen chapter 8, The Secret Treatise of the Spiritual Orchid.

Ling shu chapter 8, Ben Shen, is a strong call for the stability of the *shen*, spirits, to be central to every treatment.

Not failing to observe the four seasons and adapting to cold and heat, harmonising elation and anger, and being calm at rest as in action, regulating yinyang and balancing the hard and the soft. In this way, having removed perverse influences, there will be long life and lasting vision.

Within its traditional structure of the Emperor's question followed by the Minister's reply, this chapter contains an important discussion of 13 successive terms and their interrelationship. This book focuses on this particular section of the text and is effectively a workbook that allows the reader access to the characters of the original text itself. The 13 terms roll on like a waterfall and are taken slowly, line by line, character by character, to present the weave and pattern of the cloth as much as the individual threads themselves. These terms are key to a deeper understanding of Chinese medicine with their strong connection to our mental, emotional and spiritual nature: *de*, virtue; *qi, sheng*, life; *jing*, essences; *shen*, spirits; *hun; po; xin*, heart; *yi*, intent; *zhi*, will; *si*, thought; *lü*, reflection; *zhi*, wisdom.

Central to this series is the heart, pivot between the spiritual and mental faculties, calm seat of the emotions. Empty, to receive, unobstructed, to allow the free flow of life on every level. Here the *wu shen*, the five spiritual aspects: *shen, hun, po, yi, zhi*, are studied in depth and in context of the whole chapter. This is a profound text, constructed with the simple lightness of the Dao de jing, illustrating the clarity and depth of perception apparent at the time and no less necessary to the modern practitioner.

Claude Larre and Elisabeth Rochat de la Vallée, of the Ricci Institute and European School of Acupuncture in Paris, are both lecturers of international repute who have helped to preserve the vitality and depth of Chinese thought with their special blend of scholarship, perception and humour. They bring to Chinese medicine all the benefits of their long-term study of Chinese culture and thinking in general and their deep and detailed knowledge of the Daoist texts in particular, shedding light on what can, without guidance, seem obscure, abstruse or confused, giving the feel of the Chinese perspective as much as the actual words themselves.

Following questions arising from the text is a discussion of dreams and the emotions and an excerpt from Guanzi Neiye, The Art of the Heart, a non-medical text which again emphasizes the leading nature of the heart, calm centre of life.

When a man is capable of being correct and quiescent, his flesh is full, his ears and eyes sharp and clear, his muscles taut, and his bones sturdy. Thus he is able to wear on his head the great circle (of Heaven) and tread on the great square (of Earth).

A special feature of this Monkey Press book is the presentation the Chinese text in the most user-friendly way to give maximum access to any reader, assuming no previous knowledge of Chinese whatever. In the book itself the text of Ling shu chapter 8 is discussed line by line. For each line the characters are presented, reading from above down within the line and from right to left across the page. The transliteration in *pin yin* is also given, enabling each character to be identified with ease. In addition the main body of the text is given at the back of the book. This is provided in a pull-out form so that the text can be viewed alongside the discussion of each individual line. The text is divided into different sections to present a clear picture of the structure and with each line clearly numbered. A translation is also given. This workbook style allows a greater understanding of the Chinese perspective on life which necessarily underlies Chinese medicine, thereby enriching both study and practice.

Peter Firebrace January 1991

FOREWORD TO THE SECOND EDITION

In his original foreword to The Heart, Peter Firebrace spoke of its 'workbook' quality. This was a helpful observation and having turned to the book many times over the years since its first publication, that sense of it being an invaluable resource and study aid for the essential concepts of Chinese medicine has not diminished. Chapter 8 of the Ling shu contains a very clear statement and discussion of 13 key terms in Chinese medicine along with the role of the heart as a necessary central void and pivot which enables all else to flow freely around it.

Father Larre and Elisabeth Rochat de la Vallée have always emphasized the need for a firm foundation in the classical texts, and this book more than any other in the series of Chinese Medicine from the Classics, allows the reader to feel an intimate connection with each individual Chinese character as they are explained and seen to chain together through the text creating one of the most simple yet illuminating presentations of ancient Chinese medical philosophy.

While many readers and students search for textbooks which are immediately applicable to daily practice in the treatment room, this book stands as a companion to The Secret Treatise of the Spiritual Orchid (reissued in 2003). They are works of interpretation and explanation which give a philosophical framework for our understanding of Chinese medicine. The main thrust of chapter 8 of the Ling shu is that in our own lives and in our treatments we must root ourselves in the spirits, and by studying this translation and commentary that is precisely what we are doing.

Although, as we progress with this series, we may attempt to make the language more accessible, it is not our intention to create a perfect English rendition. It is important to keep in mind that this is the transcript of a seminar, given by two people whose first language is French. As Father Larre once pointed out, this may appear to be a problem, but in fact it gives us the opportunity to question our use of language, to question some of those literary habits and things we take for granted. Their work is not merely an attempt to translate and explain, but to allow the mind to engage with the concepts, to question and fathom and turn the ideas around in the mind until they form something new.

We have referred to Dr. L. Weiger's Chinese Characters, published by Dover Publications Inc., New York (ISBN 486 21321 8). This book is an invaluable resource for the etymology, history and meaning of Chinese characters.

Caroline Root and Sandra Hill 2004

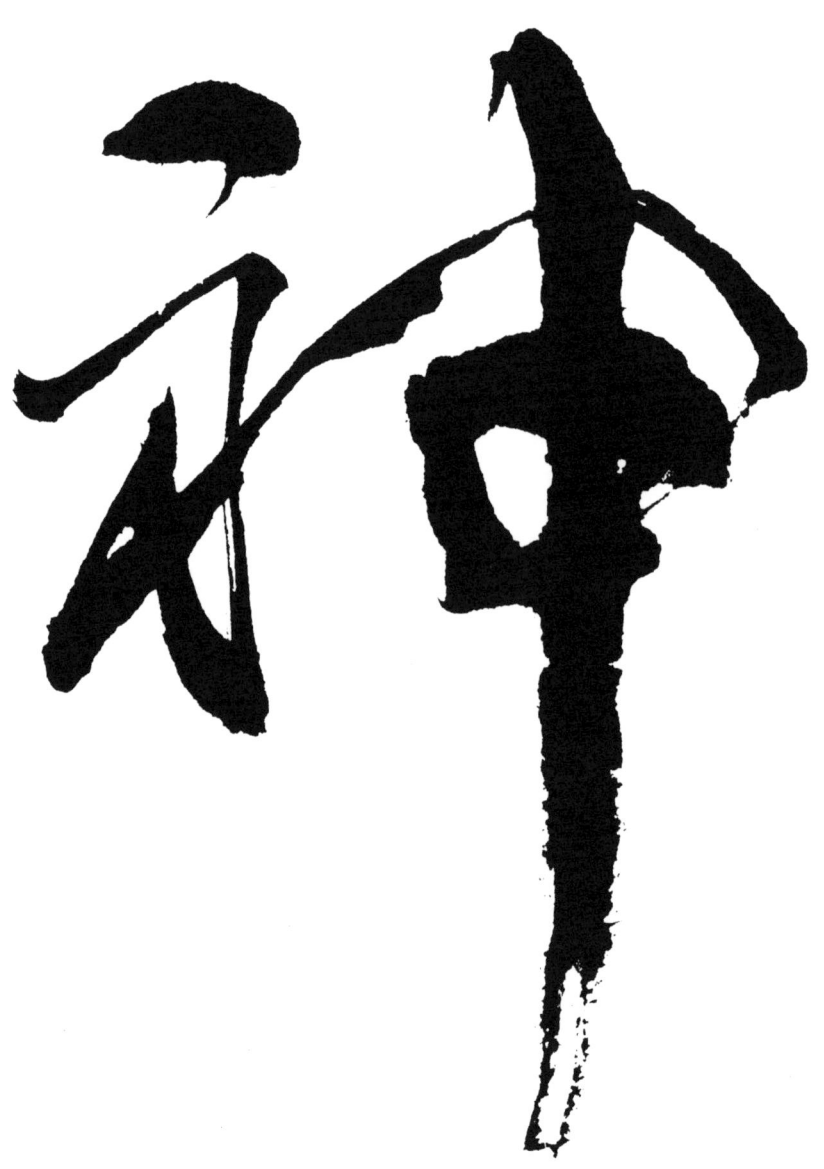

shen 神 spirits

INTRODUCTION

Claude Larre: Ling shu chapter 8 presents so much material which is so inter-connected, that we need to have a general view of how this terminology is explained in the mind of the Chinese. The best way is to look at this chapter in the same way that we looked at chapter 8 of the Su wen, where we were able to see how the internal organs or officials were working together. [cf. The Secret Treatise of the Spiritual Orchid, originally published by Monkey Press in 1985, 3rd edition published 2003]

It is very common for commentators on the classical texts to refer to these two chapters, and my feeling is that the number eight is significant in itself. Perhaps it means that it is appropriate to organise the inner life through this pattern of eight. We can see the same thing in embryology where we are working with the extraordinary meridians, and there we also find eight. The winds in the universe are made from dispersion and reunion, and are classified under this number eight. And since we know that the winds are just another name for *qi* (氣), when taken within the general pattern of heaven and earth, we understand this organisation by eight to be the primitive organisation of life. It is also the number of the *ba gua* (八 卦), the eight trigrams.

Although numerology is not our subject, we have to keep in mind that there can be no understanding of the way the Chinese explain the interplay of the internal organs and indeed every other component of life without referring to numerology. But we never take this numerology as an intellectual game. We would prefer to say that we are beings living within so many circles of life and that the development of life can be seen through different stages which are affected by number. The unity of life is something that we feel so intimately that when we feel the integration of our life with the life of another person or with the general life of others, we feel it is a healthy condition, a joyful condition, because life enjoys the same thing. And what it enjoys is this unity.

So numerology is nothing other than to be absorbed in the movement of life and to try to explain to our minds how it works. It is some sort of process; not a dry arithmetic of numbers, but the flux of life - an abstract expression of something which is absolutely concrete and real. It remains a mystery and a problem that we should be able, just from the resources of our own minds, to put so much order into life around us that we can express the core of its being. This of course is what all philosophers try to do. We ourselves are concerned with the same problems as Plato or Descartes: what is the right method by which to understand what we are doing here in this universe? We know that the Chinese, being very attached to the study of life, were as concerned as we are with the problem 'What does that mean?' and 'What am I supposed to do?', or 'What am I supposed to understand in order to shine some sort of light on my life that I may be able to get on with it?'

The Chinese way of ordering the mind is not the same as the European way of thinking since it is expressed through a special language, the ideomatic language. They have a particular view of things and the relationship between those things, rather than a way of reasoning. I am not saying that the Chinese are not thinkers or that they are not able to have structures of logical opposition; they are able to do that, but the so-called computing system is built into the characters, so a good knowledge of the Chinese text implies a true understanding of each of the characters within the systematic organisation of two, four, six or eight of them which make a full sentence.

Faced with the Chinese text, we are supposed to know the meaning of each of the characters as exactly as possible. But more than that, we have to feel how each of the characters is an expression of a particular movement of life, how one succeeds another, and how with this movement one to another a general pattern of life is shown. That is what we have to do. And that is the reason why we depend on the text.

We take for granted that you know the general approach of acupuncture from your practice and from your training at the different colleges, and we come just to contribute the knowledge of the text. In Paris we established The European School of Acupuncture, but actually, the more we progress, the more we feel we have a school for the study of the texts. We want to be known for preserving the texts and trying to draw more enlightenment from them, not to replace or to change, but just to put what people understand and what they are doing in a clearer light.

We have chosen chapter 8 of the Ling shu because in our work we find that we always come back to the same chapters. There are 81 chapters in the Ling shu, in the Su wen, in the Nan jing and in the Lao zi. But in certain chapters the systematic presentation is so well co-ordinated that knowing a short section of certain chapters well gives an additional insight which may be used everywhere.

THE CHARACTERS FOR LING SHU

Elisabeth Rochat: We will start with this chapter, Ling shu chapter 8, *ben shen* (本 神). But first let us take a look at the characters *ling shu* (靈 樞) which form the name of the second part of the Nei jing. *Ling* (靈) represents the influences that fall from above like rain. The lower section depicts three people who are exclaiming and asking for rain, the squares are three mouths [cf. Wieger, Chinese Characters, Lesson 72K].

INTRODUCTION • 5

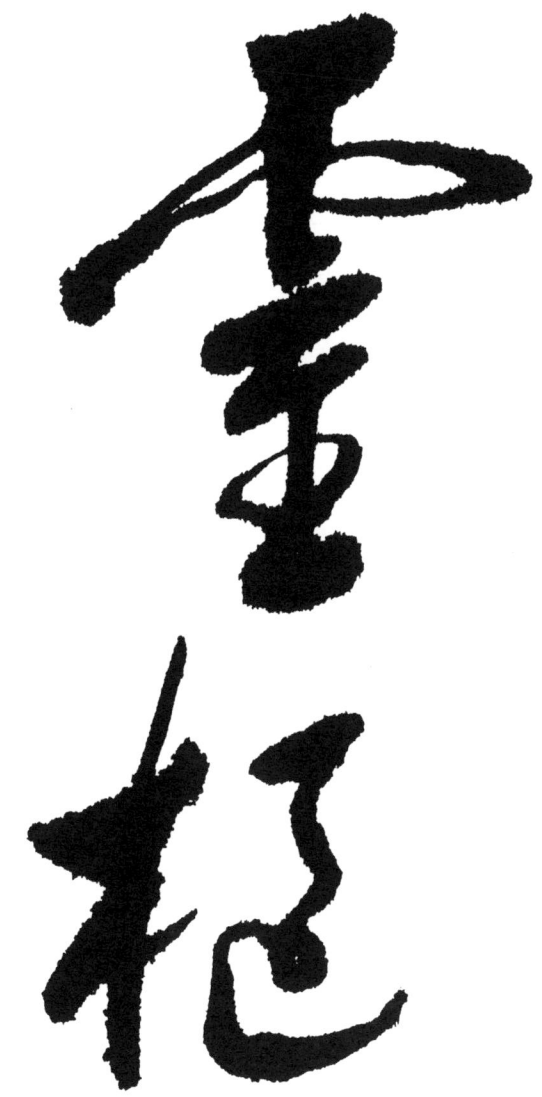

Ling shu 靈樞

Most often *ling* (靈) implies an influence that is received from heaven, or from the spirits, *shen* (神). *Ling* are terraces or places that are raised up, and it is to these places that you go to observe heaven, to receive influences from heaven, or to get yourself in a good condition to receive the influences of heaven. If you receive heavenly influences but are not capable of understanding and containing them, then that will do more harm than good. So within this character is the suggestion that there has to be a good correspondence between what is given and what is received.

In the second character, *shu* (樞), there is the idea of a pivot, something between opening and closing, with the idea of moving from opening to closing and closing to opening.

Claude Larre: And it is also like a revolving door - the entrance and the exit are circling around a pivot.

Elisabeth Rochat: We know that before being called the Ling shu, this collection of chapters within the Nei jing was called The Classic of the Needles, or The Needle Classic. There are other older names as well, but they all revolve around this notion of the needle. The first chapter of the Ling shu, which is called The Nine Needles and the Twelve Sources, describes the action of these nine needles. Throughout the Ling shu there are other chapters which deal with needles, which seems to indicate that the name Ling shu could also refer to the needle, in that the needle can be like an intermediary or pivot which allows opening and closing and communication, and once this communication is established then the influences can move through. They can pass between the doctor and the patient, or perhaps the doctor is just a pivot like the needle. At that moment the celestial influences, which are called *ling,* (the power of life, the power of heaven,) can return once more to the patient. This power of heaven can penetrate the patient through the intermediary, and this is what is necessary to re-establish an equilibrium that has been disturbed.

A human being is endowed with reason and reflection, and contains the most subtle spirits that exist on earth, and any disturbance will go to that which is most subtle and most refined. And the most subtle things are the spirits. Spirits (*shen* 神) is a character that can be used very generally to indicate everything that is the power of life in a human being, but which is without form. Spirits barely even have the form of *qi.* Everything that has form, which can be touched or seen, allows us to see what is behind that form.

Chapter 47 of the Ling shu, *ben zang* (本 臟), describes in great detail the appearance of each of the organs or *zang.* Chapter 2 of the Ling shu is called *ben shu* (本 輸). It is not the same *shu* as in Ling shu, but another which has the meaning of *shu* or transporting point. A *shu* point is not very visible or sensitive - but you have to be sensitive to it.

Claude Larre: There is nothing to be seen and it is difficult to make any association with what we know. But there is a knowledge of it, so it is a very non-material thing that we are looking for. That is the idea of the point which is conveyed by the Chinese character *shu*. In other words when you touch the body in a certain place you expect that something will happen, and that the patient will feel better. To feel better means that some part of the body is echoing what you are doing, and that from this place where you have been needling a flux is sent or is moved to another part. It is the feeling of going from one place to another that is built into the character *shu* (輸), because on the left side of the character is a chariot for transportation and the other part is two boats floating alongside each other. This means that what we are doing here is making a parallel effect on the flux of life. Your action is received and the person's life goes through some sort of transportation accordingly. That is the meaning of *shu*.

Elisabeth Rochat: The three chapters follow the same pattern, *ben shu*, chapter 2, *ben shen*, chapter 8, *ben zang*, chapter 47, and they suggest a triple rooting - in the points, in the spirits and in the internal organs. If the *zang* (臟) represent the dwelling place of the spirits, and if the spirits are the secret animation of the *zang*, then spirits and *zang* are like heaven and earth. Thus, the points on the human body represent the activity, the sensitivity, in the median, and perhaps the way to re-establish the relationship between spirits and *zang*.

THE CHARACTERS FOR BEN SHEN

Claude Larre: To come back to the meaning of *shen* (神), the presence of heaven within me is given by the *shen* flocking down to rest in me. The general feeling of *shen* is vague, celestial, intangible and all that - but the *shen* are really connected with each individual part of my body. It is difficult for us to understand because we have two contrary concepts, one is *shen* at large, and the other is *shen* operating specifically here and there. Later on we will be able to see how to connect different perceptions of the same mysterious fact, that the action is celestial and brought to us by the *shen* coming from heaven and falling down upon us, resting somewhere and being able to move our life through a certain process which will be described step by step, and each step will be specified by a different character.

I just want to warn you against too universal an idea of *shen* without a corresponding effect on the body, or against an appreciation of *shen* which is so connected with the body that the celestial power is not correctly understood. The fact is that we are working from one concept to another, and that is the ordinary way that our minds work. But the Chinese are not doing that, they are just writing characters, and through the characters we have to see how many different lines of perception are offered. *Shen* is offering the view of heavenly effect. At the same time *shen* is giving you an indication of the most precise ways to move the *qi* either in yourself or in a patient.

The character *ben* (本) from *ben shen*, is composed with the radical number 75, *mu* (木), with the meaning of tree or wood. It is quite obvious that this character is one of the five elements, wood as an element and more concretely, a tree. Wood as a material is not wood as an element. Wood as a material is wood to make chairs and tables. Wood as an element is a kind of vibration. We know that the wind, the wood, the green colour, the acid taste and the muscles are different stages in that vibration or resonance; wind is known by its producing force, but wood is known by its fibre, and muscle is known by its fibre. Acid is known by its progressive mode, and the green colour is the colour of grass, trees and all sorts of growing plants. They are growing up progressively and they are bending, and going everywhere. That is all part of the same aspect of life which is encompassed by this character *mu* (木).

But the Chinese way to use this radical is to fix the central idea and then to make further division and clarification. We might be interested in the part of the tree where the trunk is penetrating the earth with different roots, so to mark that part of the character which is specifically indicated we draw a small line. Then we are indicating that within this character we choose one specific aspect of the tree which is the root and the trunk. Each of us is able to live because we are well rooted, and because we are well rooted,

INTRODUCTION • 11

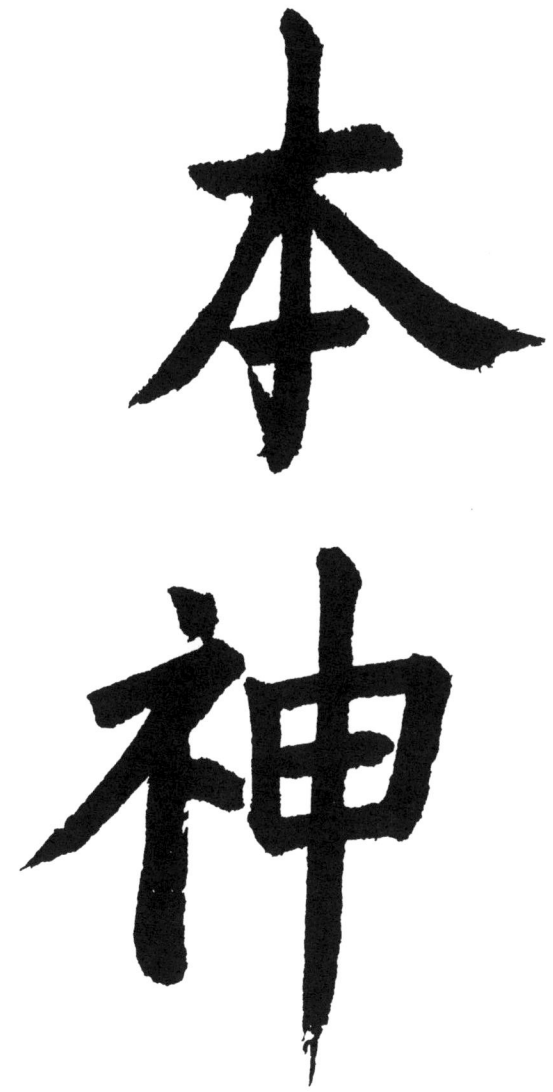

ben shen 本 神

we are able to spring up vertically like a plant. But, another time, we may be interested in the top of the character, which, with one extra stroke on top, becomes an ear of corn, (mo 末). So we can play with this radical, doubling it we have two trees, a lot of trees, a wood, (lin 林). Or perhaps three of them, and that would be a forest (sen 森). So when we look at a character, we do not only consider the meaning which is given in the dictionary for the first word of the first line, because there are so many meanings which are compatible with the character and it is connecting all these circles with the other circles given by the following character, and it is really the whole line which makes the context in which the word itself has to be seen.

There is always much more in the Chinese text than in the English text, since the visible aspect of the character enriches the meaning of what is presented. It is difficult to understand the guiding line of the expression with so many significations moving between the characters. But in Chinese as in any other language, we look at the end. If someone starts to speak, you understand that they are attempting to get somewhere and there is more meaning at the end than in the middle part or at the beginning. At the beginning there is strength, the approach to the subject is usually very clear and very bright, and it goes step by step to the end.

With the trunk and the root, the two associated meanings are that the trunk needs the roots and the roots express themselves to form this well built body of life, which is something very close to another aspect of the tree, which is the stem. Stems and branches have something to do with this idea of *ben* (本) or *mu* (木). The branches are the lateral expression, but the stem is the vertical expression. The stem is standing but does not give the same impression as *ben*. *Ben* is insisting on the root which is a trunk, which is not the case with stem. You can see from this very simple example, that when it is the same English or French word which is used to make a translation referring to a stage where the expression is still Chinese and not yet English, you have to feel how life presents itself, and you keep that in mind.

Now let us come to *shen*. *Shen* (神) is made with two parts. The left part (示) is radical number 113, which has something to do with spirits. The spirits are not seen directly, but there is the image of somebody making a sacrifice and arranging a table with a stand from which something will rise. The right hand part is made from a primitive form of writing in which one part of the influence is going one way and the other part is going the other way. So the concept and impression given by *shen* is of an influx developing in both directions. And that influence is immaterial, not in the sense that it is non-substantial, it is not a question of logic. It is just that you cannot see it, but you may receive it, and you may feel it. You can see it in your patients, when the patient is in a better condition, you can feel it, and he or she feels it. Everything is restored to life, and that is the effect of the spirits. It may be visible on the face, in the emission from the eyes, the brightness of the face, the smile, the alertness, everything is so active, so many spirits are moving that life is now restored. And this is the meaning of the radiance of the *shen*. Radiance is perceptible, and if something is perceptible it is because something is working. The spirit is shown through the radiance: there would be no radiance without something to irradiate.

So the character *ben* (本) is insisting that you have to go to the roots of life, and *shen* (神) that you have to move the lazy *shen*, or to call the *shen* back because they may be displeased with the state of the disorder where they are supposed to rest. If they have no place to rest they will not stay. And *ben shen* for the physician or for the therapist is to go with knowledge and power into that place and try to move something, to attract the spirits and make them work again.

Elisabeth Rochat: It is also interesting to see that in the primitive characters for the spirits there is the idea of an alternating power which makes life, and which within the spirits is at the same time imperceptible and indissociable, it cannot be separated. The spirits are a power which can accept everything that is *yin* (陰) as well as everything that is *yang* (陽) but they cannot be analysed according to *yin* and *yang*, they are beyond that.

This is confirmed by the Great Commentary, Xi ci, on the Yi jing, The Book of Change, where the great definition of the *shen* is that they cannot be detected through *yin* and *yang*, because reconciling the two and being at the same time beyond them, the *shen* represent the power of life in its heavenly unity, capable of penetrating and embracing, containing and accepting the *yin* and *yang* which creates life on earth.

You find spirits, *shen*, joined together with something which we consider to be very *yang*, like *qi* (氣), and also with something which we consider very *yin* like *jing* (精), essences. You find both couples, *shen qi*, *jing shen*, and the *jing qi*, essences and *qi*, themselves constitute a couple. So we have the three great key terms in Chinese medicine where the spirits represent the power of heaven, the *qi* represents the power of earth, because it is by the virtue of the *qi* that all forms are created, and the essences refer to that which is joined together in the middle. All this will be clearer when we look at the text of Ling shu chapter 8.

Claude Larre: I will just say something about *shen* and *qi*, *shen* being the leading factor and *qi* being the expression of the leading factor. Whenever we discuss *qi* we refer to *yin qi* or *yang qi*, or a mixture of *yin qi* and *yang qi*. There is no living being incorporated in the universe which is not the result of a good combination of *yin qi* and *yang qi*. The vitality of that which is neither *yin* nor *yang* is on a higher level, on the level of the spirits. Without the spirits the *yin qi* and *yang qi* are not able to turn to one another, so we have to draw a line to separate *shen* from *qi*. But the *shen* and *qi* together make the term *shen qi* (神 氣), which is the expression of life drawn by the *qi* under the guidance of the *shen*. This is a more *yang* aspect, because *qi* as vitality refers to the more lively aspect of ourselves. *Jing* refers to the more *yin* aspect, because it is impossible to have any vitality without a very strong basis for it.

When you assimilate various kinds of food, you build the same thing in yourself, in your essences, and from these essences you will be able to manifest the spirits which are working within you. The spirits from heaven are your own spirits, but they are your own only because of the specific pattern which is given by the essences. The combination of essences and spirits give *jing shen* (精 神), which is more like the vitality of life.

The three main characters, *shen* (神), *qi* (氣) and *jing* (精) are now in place. These are the characters that are linked at the beginning of the Ling shu.

THE TEXT

The following is a discussion of the first section of the text of Ling shu chapter 8 taken line by line. The Chinese characters are presented reading from above to below within the line and from right to left across the page.

In addition, the main body of the text is given at the back of the book. This is provided in a pull-out form so that the text can be viewed alongside the discussion of each individual line. The text is divided into different sections to present the reader with a clear picture of the text's structure, with each line clearly numbered. An English translation is also given. In this way no previous knowledge of Chinese is necessary to gain maximum benefit from the text and commentary.

THE EMPEROR'S QUESTION

line 1: *huang di wen yu qi bo ye*
line 2: *fan ci zhi fa*
   xian bi ben yu shen

黃帝問於歧伯曰
凡刺之法先必本于神

Elisabeth Rochat: The very beginning of chapter 8 is a question from Huangdi, the Emperor, to his minister about the method of needling, *ci zhi fa* (刺 之 法).

Claude Larre: The *ci* (刺) character has the knife on the right side. It is not exactly a knife, but it has the same effect of piercing the skin. The left hand part suggests a thorn. So this character has something to do with thorns and the effect of pricking and entering the flesh. *Zhi* (之) is a general character for linking, and *fa* (法) is the method.

The sentence continues:

xian bi ben yu shen
先 必 本 于 神

Bi is not to be confused with heart. *Bi* (必) is almost the same as the character for heart, *xin* (心), with one additional slanting stroke. It means necessary, it is necessary, it has to be, and so on, and sometimes it just reflects that things are how they are, so it is difficult to put an additional English word, just be content with the necessity of it!

The character *xian* (先) is not very interesting etymologically. We have to separate the issues, some characters are more important than others. *Ben* (本) is the root. *Yu* (于) means to go towards, it has no special etymology, and *shen* (神) is the spirits. It is necessary to go to the roots to reach the spirits.

This means that it is not just the location that is important, not just the points that you needle. Of course, you have to know what you are doing, but you must keep in mind that you have to wait for the right time and for the right condition when these spirits, which are animating the whole body, are ready to receive your attention. They will receive it through the *qi*. The spirits are never separated from the *qi* but you have to recall the spirits through the *qi*. Moving the *qi* you will be able to change the condition of the mind, and from that change, the flow of life will be corrected. There will be no more *xie qi* (邪 氣), perverse *qi,* but *zheng qi* (正 氣), the normal or correct *qi.*

To do that you will have to put your mind in phase with your patient's mind. Not mind in the meaning of intellectual mind, but mind in the more profound, more comprehensive meaning. This individual, after all, is a person, and you are a person, it is a personal exchange. Help is possible if you reach to the spirits. If you do not reach the spirits you may have a temporary good effect, but it will be destroyed soon after. But if you have moved life where it is built through the spirits, then these changes will stay for as long as the condition is good enough for the spirits to stay. So it is interesting to understand that some sort of metaphysics is necessary. That is the reason why I myself am engaged in this business, not to cure, but to understand whether or not the Chinese had some sort of understanding of life which encompasses the interaction of individuals. It is in a sphere which is not intellectual, it is some sort of spiritual life.

But is it the field of acupuncture or not? We can be sure that according to the way of their own civilization, the Chinese did not restrict what they were doing to the *qi.* They were going further, and that has to be the *shen.* And that is the reason why we have to be comfortable with this, because it is from our knowledge of the spirits that we are able to cure people for good.

line 3: *xue mai ying qi jing shen
ci wu zang zhi suo cang ye*

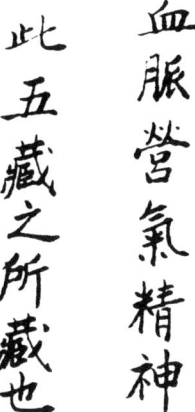

Elisabeth Rochat: The Emperor starts his question with an affirmation when he says that in every case when you needle you have to go to the root of the spirits. This is something that he has received and already knows. Then he passes to another affirmation which is the following: *xue mai* (血 脈), *ying qi* (營 氣), *jing shen* (精 神), are all stored in and through the five *zang* (臟). So we have a very clear first construction: a rooting in the spirits. And we know that these spirits can embrace all that exists. Immediately following this we have the vitality functioning through these six terms, and their storing or keeping preciously by the five *zang*.

These six terms represent three couples. It is easy to see that *jing shen* (精 神), essences and spirits, form a couple, and you can see that *xue mai* (血 脈) is another couple which is frequently seen in the Nei jing. *Ying* (營), nutrition, and *qi* (氣), is another couple which represents vitality. In each couple there is a *yin* and a *yang* aspect. The blood, *xue* (血), is the *yin* aspect and the *mai* (脈) is the *yang* aspect. It is the same for the second couple; the nutrition, *ying*, is a deeper, more nourishing aspect in contrast with the *qi*, especially if we take *qi* as the defensive or *wei qi* (衛氣). And finally our last couple *jing shen* (精 神), the essences give a substance which is *yin*, in relationship to the *shen*.

Question: Can I ask about the *shen* because sometimes it is described as neither *yin* nor *yang* but encompasses both, and sometimes it is seen as very *yang*?

Claude Larre: Yin and *yang* are not to be used absolutely. They have to be used contextually. The context is that there are three couples, one matching *xue* and *mai*, another matching *ying* and *qi*, and a third, *jing* and *shen* which refers to mankind. You may feel that *jing shen* is more *yang*, but it is impossible that this *yang* dynamism would not be resting on some *yin* power, which is the essences. So, even if the *jing shen* gives you the impression that the *yang* is dominating, you are just looking at the *yang* aspect of the *jing shen*. It is sure that *yin yang* may play as an expression in our minds more freely than any other because it is the highest combination.

Elisabeth Rochat: If we look at the first couple, *xue mai* (血

脈), we see that there is a movement of pushing and circulation. The richness of life is represented by the blood, and we will see that the blood is full of *jing*, essences, and *shen*, spirits, because the blood holds the spirits. There is a movement of animation, of pushing forwards, which is represented by the *mai*, whose power is both to push forward and to keep within limits.

In the second couple, *ying qi* (營 氣), we find all the power of nutrition, *ying*, the maintenance of life by alimentation and the *qi*, that permits the circulation and defence of the body. There is something that spreads everywhere rhythmically in the *qi*.

In the last couple, *jing shen* (精 神) we have the most subtle, most refined expression of this vitality, with the composition and harmonious re-composition, of everything that makes up the individual being; the *jing*, essences, which serve as a support for the action of the spirits. Their action is just to be, and to be present. And with the presence of the *jing shen* there is a manifestation of brilliance, which is the radiance that Father Larre was talking about.

If we look again at these characters, we see that blood is linked with the liver, and the *mai* (脈) with the heart. This is exactly what is stated right at the end of this chapter of the Ling shu. Everything that involves nutrition, *ying*, is linked with the spleen, the *qi* is linked with the lung, and the essences, *jing*, are those of the kidneys. Then there are just the spirits, and of course we know that the spirits reside in the heart. We have, as so often in the Nei jing, a double presence which can be linked with either the kidneys or the heart. Here it is the double presence of the heart which will enlighten us on the two aspects of the heart.

If we look now at the names of the meridians which are attributed to these various organs, we see that in the middle couple, *ying qi*, we have the two sides of *tai yin* (太 陰), the lung and the spleen meridians, and in the third couple, *jing shen*, we have the two sides of *shao yin* (少 陰), the kidney and heart meridians. So we may wonder if at the beginning, *xue mai*, we are not faced with the two sides of *jue yin* (厥 陰), the liver and heart master meridians?

Almost certainly - since we know that the heart has a double meridian, and that the heart has a double presentation. The heart is either a void which allows the spirits to dwell within or else it is that activity which allows the spirits to circulate and the heart to exercise its authority as governor or master. It exercises its authority especially over all the vital circulations, *mai* (脈), through which the blood particularly is circulated. We will come back to the different links of the blood with the heart, liver, spleen and so on. We will just say that through this network for vital animation which is the *mai*, we can see the *qi* and blood circulate.

But you can also say, as it is indeed said in Ling shu chapter 8, that the *mai* are the dwelling place of the spirits, just as it is said that the heart is the dwelling place of the spirits. The heart itself is a void or place of quietness for the spirits. Another aspect of the heart is the presence of the effect of the spirits everywhere in the body through the blood or the *qi*, the aspect is that of circulating, of sending out, and of reaching everywhere.

This is just a first insight into this aspect of the heart as a void which we will develop later. But it is fundamental to understanding how these six terms are arranged even in such an ordinary or commonly used series as this.

The chapter goes on to say that all these six are stored in and through the five *zang* (臟). All these couples are an expression of a vitality which is itself an expression of *yin yang*. All this is in a permanently changing movement, and it is because of this that the *zang* appear. The *zang* are governed by the number five, not six. The five *zang* represent the five different movements whose changes and interpenetration permit life to take place. It is through these five movements that life takes place. And it is through the void that the movement is expressed.

So there can only be five centres of attraction, five poles within the body, and there can only be five *zang*, even if they are sometimes counted as six or nine or twelve. We are looking at the fundamental constitution of life, and there can only be five. All life takes place between five and six. Five represents the animation, the communication, the compenetration of these different movements. Six the maintenance and the animation of life, everything that ensures that life can carry on, that life can be made, re-made and maintained. There are other lists of six terms in the Ling shu where we can see the same thing, and if we analyse and differentiate we always have to remember that it is the totality of them that makes the whole being. The role of the spirits, relying on the essences, is perhaps to guarantee this unity of life at every moment, this unity that can be divided up into all these different terms.

We can carry on looking at many different combinations between these six. For example we can look at the *sheng* (生) cycle, the cycle of production, from liver (*xue*, blood) to heart (*mai*), heart to spleen (*ying*, nutrition), spleen to lung (*qi*), and lung to kidney (*jing*, essences). And after the kidney to the void centre of the spirits (*shen*).

Claude Larre: I would just like to add something about the question *ci zhi fa* (刺 之 法), the way of needling. It implies that we are concerned with the *mai* and the blood. We are concerned with the *qi* of the patient, and the *ying*, which is not only nourishing but is building and re-building that person, because *ying* has the meaning of to build. And looking at the face of the patient you feel that they have much *jing shen* or little *jing shen*. I just want to stress that it is with reference to the needling process that those general statements are made. So why do they start with *xue mai?* Perhaps because it is question of *ci zhi fa.* And why do they come here? Perhaps because it is a question of whether or not there is enough *ying qi* in that person. Why is this? Because in contrast to the *ying qi,* you should pay attention to the *jing shen* of that person. Even if we are giving an explanation of the characters in a broad general application to understand the relationship between the six, we must remain in the context of needling.

Elisabeth Rochat: There is a lot to be gained for diagnosis in this; diagnosis from the state of blood and the *mai.* This can be felt on the pulse, and can be seen in the complexion in all the small capillaries close to the surface of the skin. Then the second level of the deep nutrition and animation. This is at a deeper level than the first, with all kinds of symptoms connected with nutrition or digestion or with the *qi,* or the maintaining functions of the body, the movements and rhythms, seeing if it is all going well. Then we arrive at the last level of diagnosis which is the sum of everything that has gone before, plus the brightness of the eyes, and all the intangible aspects which are not covered by the previous four. There is a way of looking at the complexion of a person, their face, which tells you about the state of the blood, the circulation, the nutrition etc. But there is in addition to this something that does not belong to that realm and which is at the level of *jing shen.*

For the true art of needling you have to go right down to this deeper level, and it is not by chance that this series ends with the *shen*, the spirits. It moves from the visible down to the invisible.

Claude Larre: I want to link what Elisabeth has said to what I suggested at the beginning. If we want to understand where the text is pointing we have to jump to the end and say that *shen* is the last character in that series. It is because the title is *ben shen* (本 神) that the *shen* cannot be without the essences in mankind, and maybe in the universe. If the universe is perfect there are not only spirits, there must be something corresponding, even in the sun or in the moon. The vital forces penetrate everywhere and we are the result of that. What is made of the moon and the sun in ourselves is seen through the *jing shen* (精 神).

There must be some essences of the sun and some essences of the moon, and fire and water and all that. Then having this *jing shen* of the universe within us - we are closer than anything on earth to the forces of the universe. It is in the *jing shen* of humanity that the best image of the universe is given, the image of force and brightness and joy and all that. But this has to rely on the four things, the *xue mai* (血 脈), and the *ying qi* (營 氣). It is impossible not to pay attention to each of the characters individually, but it is also impossible not to see them as couples!

Elisabeth Rochat: Just keep in mind these three divisions - the *jue yin*, *tai yin* and *shao yin*, and the relationship of these six terms. This particular presentation is not long enough to give a theory about *jue yin*, *tai yin* and *shao yin*, but it is just one element to keep in your mind in order to have a better comprehension of what *jue yin*, *tai yin* and *shao yin* are.

line 4: *zhi qi yin yi li zang ze jing shi*

至其淫泆離藏
則精失

When we come to the state of affairs where under the impact of shaking and diverting something from an attack of perversity, everything is full of perverse *qi* and the *zheng qi* (正氣) in turn becomes the *xie qi* (邪氣) - when we reach that condition, then something separates itself from the *zang*. There is no longer storage of the essences, *ze jing shi* (則精失), and the essences are lost.

line 5: *hun po fei yang*
line 6: *zhi yi huang luan*

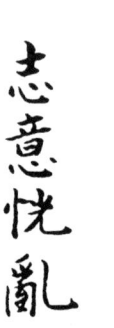

魂魄飛揚

志意恍亂

The *hun* (魂) and the *po* (魄) are going with the wind, flying and dispersing in all directions. The *zhi* (志), will power, and the *yi* (意), intent, or that which gives the will power a frame to adjust to circumstances and to make a project, that is the kidney spirits and the spleen spirits, are troubled, confused and in disorder. This means that there is no more strength and no more perception of what to do.

When we do not know what to do, when we are confused it is the *zhi* and the *yi* that are not up to dealing with a specific situation. And that comes from this first deviation. When everything is normal it is okay, but when the perverse *qi*, *xie qi* (邪氣), disturbs the equilibrium then it starts with the *zang*. They are not kept by the *shen* and they are not keeping the essences.

line 7: *zhi lü qu shen zhe*

智
慮
去
身
者

Then we move from the ultimate to the other more visible troubles. One problem that we understand very well ourselves is that if we are weak without essences, even when we want to do something we are unable to see what it is we should do, and we do not feel that we have the energy to do it. The combination of the energy with the intent (*yi* 意), or the intent with the energy is not made, and if it is not made, the mind is disturbed. When I say the mind, very often the way to explain it is that the condition of the mind is troubled: *zhi lü qu shen zhe* (智 慮 去 身 者).

The ability to act, the way that the mind is able to organise itself in order to achieve something, is no longer there. I am no longer myself, I do not feel myself. I am not only confused, I have no means to do whatever I would like to do. I am very depressed: *he yin er ran hu* (何 因 而 然 乎).

line 8: *he yin er ran hu*
tian zhi zui yu ren zhi guo hu

何因而然乎
天之罪與
人之過乎

What is the cause of it? *Tian zhi zui yu* (天 之 罪 與). Is it that heaven is responsible, or is it my fault? If it is something that is beyond my responsibility or beyond my reach, then it is heaven. Or is it that everything is correct in heaven and I am not able to respond to what heaven is presenting? Where is the fault? I am talking of responsibility. The character *zui* (罪) means that it is your fault, you are responsible. Is heaven responsible for that very poor state of affairs, or is it that you have been going astray?

I do not say that you are to blame, but the fact is that you have gone too far, exceded the limits, in one way or another. Then when disharmony is your fault, fault is seen as excess, which is not said of heaven. That is typical of Chinese classical texts. They usually say 'Is it heaven or myself who is responsible for that?' They make a distinction.

line 9: *he wei de qi sheng*
jing shen hun po
xin yi zhi si zhi lü
line 10: *qing wen qi gu*

Since this is not sufficient in itself for a question, Huangdi, who is just as keen to learn as Western acupuncturists, asks what is understood by virtue (*de* 德), *qi* (氣), life (*sheng* 生), essences (*jing* 精), spirits (*shen* 神), *hun* (魂), *po* (魄), the heart (*xin* 心), the intent (*yi* 意), the will or the direction that is given (*zhi* 志), the thought that reflects and builds itself (*si* 思), the wisdom that is know-how or the ability to do things (*zhi* 智), and the possibility of conceiving or imagining things (*lü* 慮). And he asks respectfully that he can be taught all of this!

THE MINISTER'S REPLY

line 11: *tian zhi zai wo zhe de ye*
line 12: *di zhi zai wo zhe qi ye*

天之在我者德也
地之在我者氣也

Elisabeth Rochat: Qi Bo has understood the Emperor's question so well that he is able to organise the conditions for life in a human being within the conditions of life in the universe, whether that involves the movement of the mind, the blood or the spirit. If you deviate from this movement of life, then that will produce all the catastrophes that Huangdi mentioned before. These are all examples of dissolution or decomposition, disharmony between two elements that should work together, such as the *hun* (魂) and the *po* (魄), the will, *zhi* (志), and the intent, *yi* (意), the knowledge of how to do things, *zhi* (智), and the knowledge that one can do them, *lü* (慮).

The first word in this speech by Qi Bo is heaven, *tian* (天). 'Heaven in me is virtue, earth in me is *qi*.' So here we see that the *qi* is related to the earth, and it is related to earth because the *qi* is both *yin* and *yang* in harmony and composition, alternating, and this harmony and composition of *yin* and *yang* produces all the beings that come out of the earth. This is accomplished by an impulse from heaven, the impulse from virtue, and is the way that life is produced without doing anything in particular. It is through this impulse that all the effects of life are produced. This impulse is associated with unity and the origin, associated with heaven, staying in what we call virtue in every sense of the term.

First we have the presentation of heaven, then of earth. The Chinese do not try to look at what they cannot see. They start by looking at what is in front of their eyes, and from that they try to rise to the more subtle things. If you want to find out what life is, then what is there in front of your eyes and what you can feel is your own life, and it is because of this that this pronoun *wo* (我), which means me, is there in the text. From what you can grasp of your own life you can understand what life is. If you see that within yourself there is this profound unity which goes straight forward, and that there is all this movement from the *qi* seen in various different aspects and different forms, you can see that the junction of the two, the joining of all these things will make life in one unity.

36 • THE HEART IN LING SHU 8

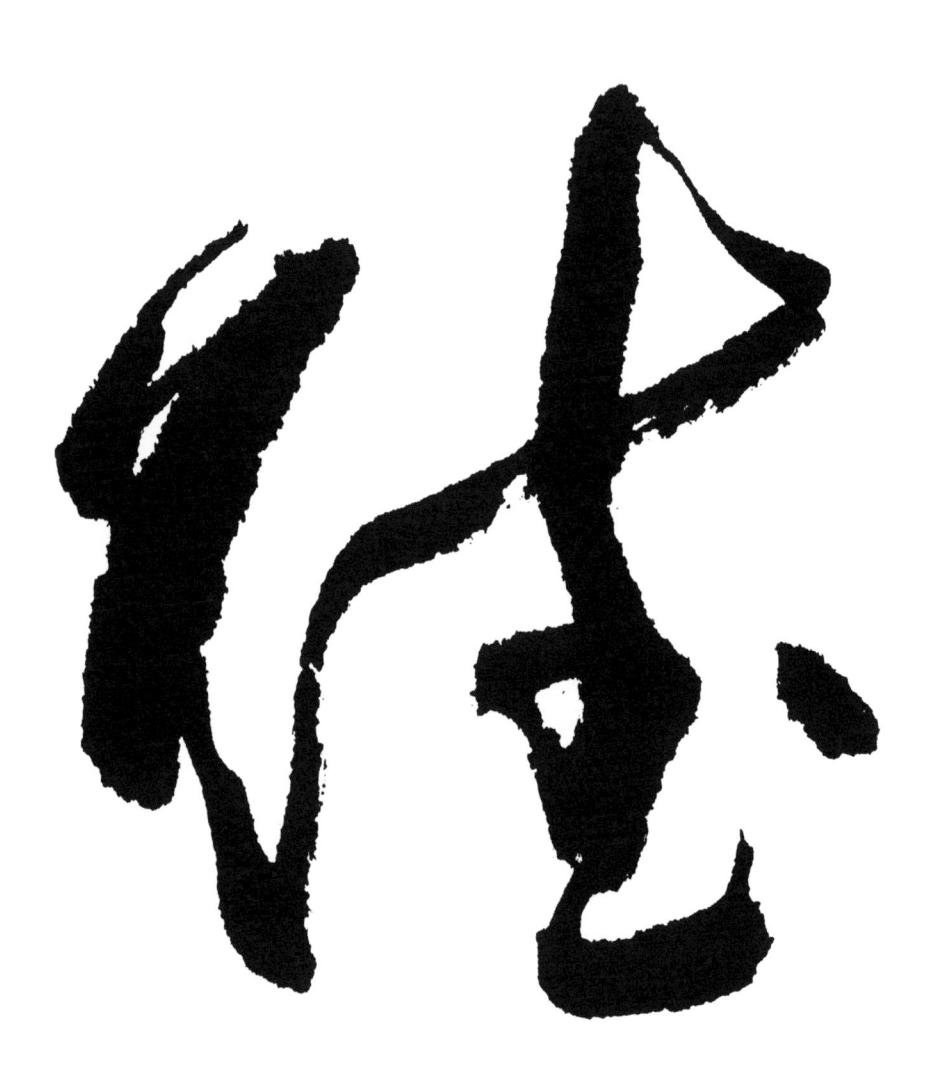

de 德 virtue

Claude Larre: He who is living has to be living because he is speaking. There is no question of am I, or am I not? To be or not to be is not the question! There is no question!

line 13: *de liu qi bo er sheng zhe ye*

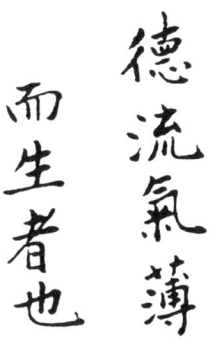

德流氣薄而生者也

Elisabeth Rochat: You can say that virtue flows, *qi* spreads everywhere, and that is what makes life. When virtue flows down from above, *(de liu* 德 流*)* and the *qi* spreads, *(qi bo* 氣 薄*)*, everywhere, that is life, *sheng zhe ye* (生 者 也).

Claude Larre: I would just like to go back again to the first lines:

tian zhi zai wo zhe de ye
天 之 在 我 者 德 也

When we say heaven here we understand that it is the presence of heaven, or its power in myself, that is alluded to. Then how do I qualify this power of heaven in myself?

38 • THE HEART IN LING SHU 8

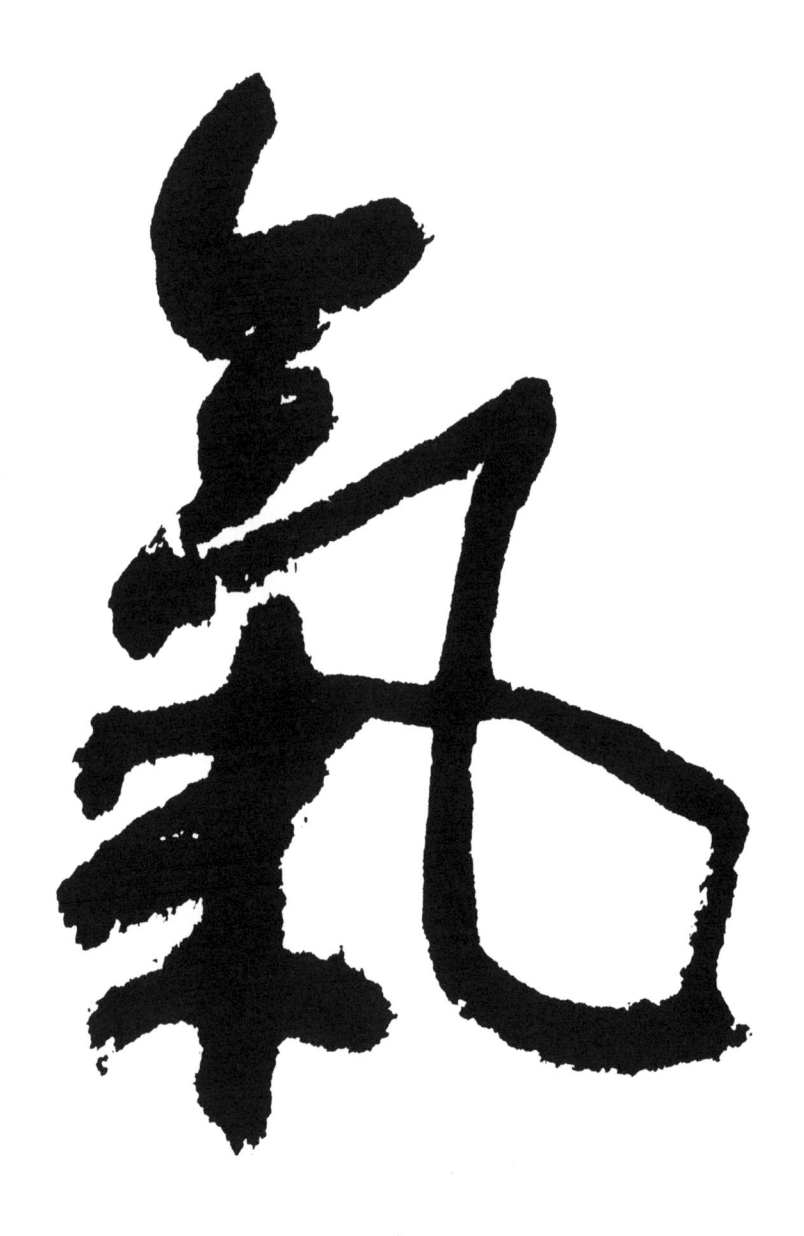

qi 氣

This is myself, *wo* (我), not in the meaning of a human being but this specific human being that I am - me, and not another. *Zhe* (者) is just insisting on making myself more evident, more objective. *De ye* (德 也), this virtue, has in our occidental mind a double meaning which makes a single meaning in the Chinese approach. The first meaning is that the virtue expressed in me, the fact that I am able to do or to be, is heaven. The other meaning is that when heaven wants to do something in the universe, it will do it even through the mediation of humanity. This is a much broader meaning which is not implied immediately in the text. But we know from other texts, especially Lao zi that not only the *dao* (道) and the virtue, which is very similar to the *dao*, and heaven and earth, are called great, but humanity is too.

Lao zi chapter 25 says: 'Great is the way, great is heaven, great is the earth and great also is the king'. So in the universe there are four greats and the king is one of them. This *wo* (我), which by itself is just myself, is as big as heaven, since my true self is operated through the virtue of heaven, and my virtue is never more complete and perfect than when everything in myself is following heaven's direction. Then we are able to understand that all the ordinary efficiency of life may be called back in case of disorder only if I am strong enough and clever enough, and non-interfering enough to make this gift from heaven operate again in the individuality of this patient.

di zhi zai wo zhe qi ye
地 之 在 我 者 氣 也

Then, contrasting earth to heaven, going through the same characters, *zhi zai wo zhe ye*, we come to the last opposition between *de* (德), virtue coming from heaven, with the *qi* (氣) coming from earth. One way to understand *de* and *qi* might be that I feel heaven within myself as virtue and I feel the presence of the earth within myself by the fact that I am full of *qi*. More specifically, coming to the actual human being that I am, I want to know how this virtue, which is me, is operating, and I want to know what the *qi* coming from the earth has to do with the formation of this individual being that I am. And it is through the effect of *liu* (流), to flow, and through the effect of *bo* (薄), to spread.

de liu qi bo er sheng zhe ye
德 流 氣 薄 而 生 者 也

The effect of *liu* is in the virtue coming from above and spreading, and the effect of *bo* is that not only does it flow, but it falls everywhere, making the kind of milieu from which I am born. We have to know more precisely how this coming to life is achieved, not only that virtue is flowing and that *qi* is spreading, but that virtue is flowing because it pertains to heaven to make its virtue come down from above, and it is in the nature of earth to make the dispersion and spreading of virtue all around. One may say that in springtime, looking at the sky, we may feel that there is enough light to make the grass grow. That would be the vertical influence of the sky, and behind that sky I know there is heaven, which I cannot see but I understand to be represented by sky.

Sky is the normal representation for heaven, it is not the same thing but it is the true image of heaven. At the same time I know that at the right moment, when it is possible that the virtue of heaven makes life appear through the sprouting of vegetation and so on, there is another complementary virtue of earth which makes sure that the vegetation will shoot up and grow. Then the horizontal or the spreading effect of the living being would be demonstrated through the virtue which is proper to earth. But this is not called virtue, which is appropriate to heaven, but *qi*. So in that context, *qi* is the natural effect of the earth, and virtue is the natural effect of heaven. And the combination of them both is what makes a living being - or what makes a being live.

Then after this description of virtue and of *qi* and the combination of heavenly virtue and earthly *qi*, are the *sheng zhe* (生者), the living beings. So how can we analyse more specifically the constituent factors of this particular individual life? I want to know within myself if there is another aspect describing the fact that I am a living being.

42 • THE HEART IN LING SHU 8

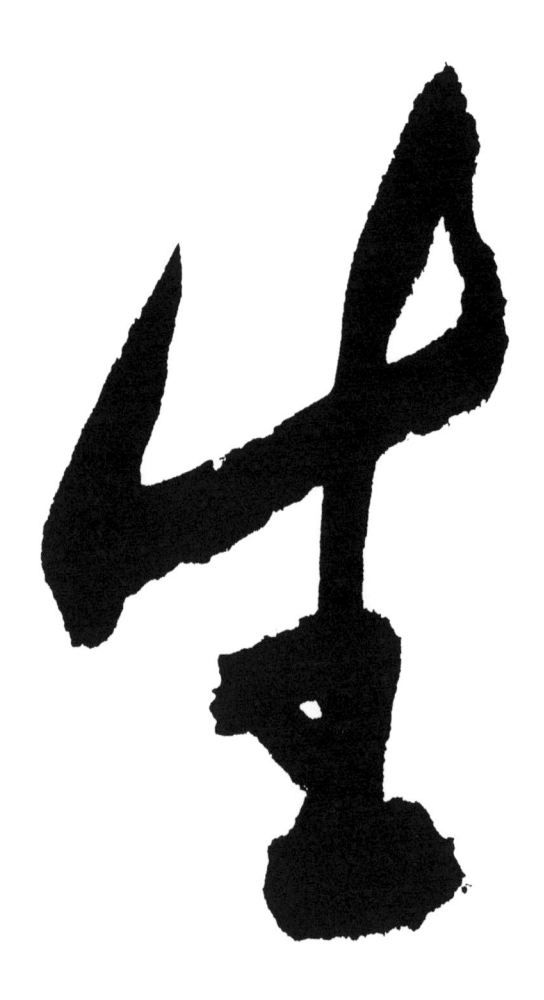

sheng 生 life

line 14: *gu sheng zhi lai wei zhi jing*

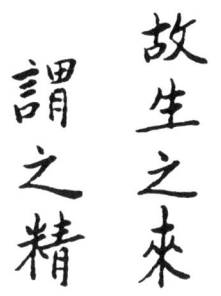

故生之來
謂之精

Then the text says: Well, as for life, when something is coming forth, then we have to have a name for this, and we call it *jing* (精).

So we need to look more closely and try to understand this; why life is coming forth, why this coming forth is called essences, and why it is pertaining to life. Then it will become clear that there can be no specific being if the individual specification is not made by the essences. Specific and essences come to the same thing. When I say specific it is more abstract, when I say essences it is just the realisation, the bringing into matter of this abstract word. And why *lai* (來)? Because the essences are called for. When I eat lunch then this same process starts operating. It is the process of digesting the essences which are in the food and they are called for by my organism. It is impossible for me to say that it is my stomach, the stomach is just one of the factors, and it has to go along with the small intestine, the large intestine, through the blood and through all the

44 • THE HEART IN LING SHU 8

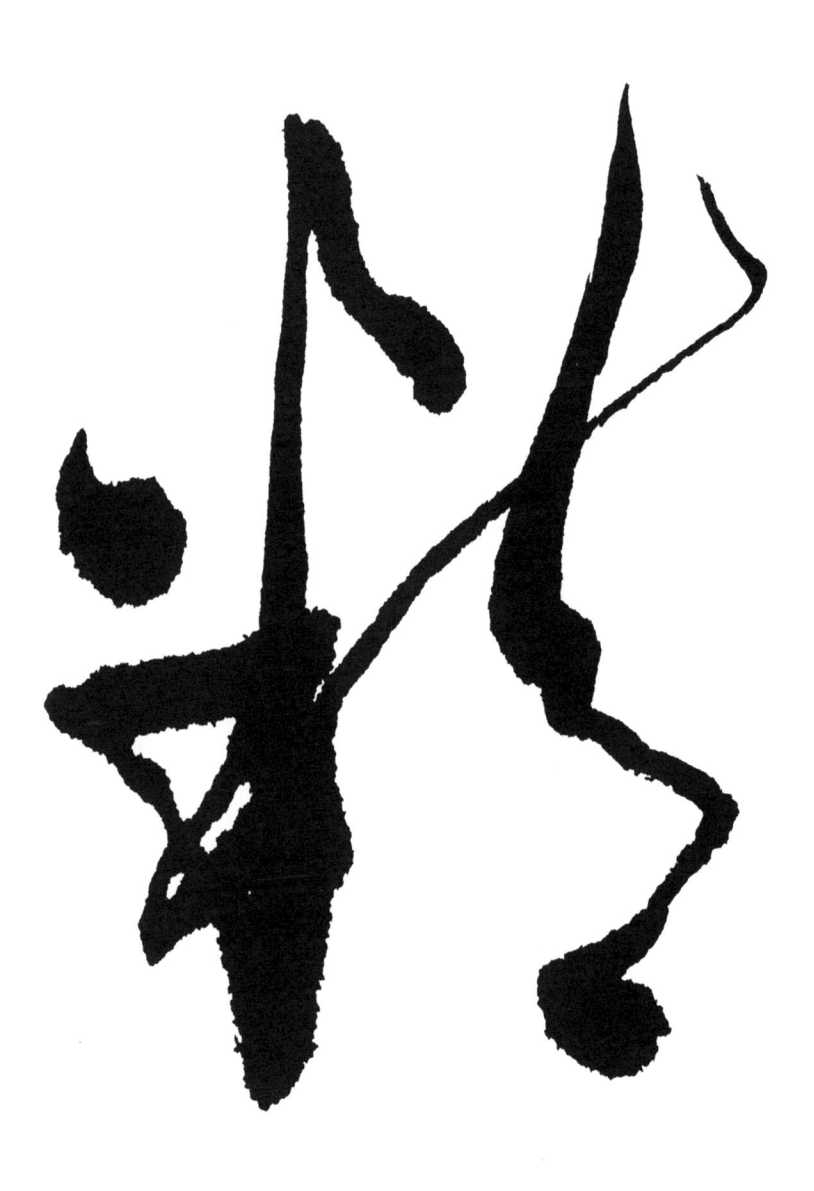

jing 精 essences

dispatching surfaces, just like in a sorting office where they sort letters and send them here and there. But this is done under the supreme control of the heart. The authority has to be completed, helped and assisted by some sort of prime minister, a counsellor to tell him how to do it, and the heart has to be defended. We can refer to Su wen chapter 8 where the twelve officials are presented. The twelve officials are those who dispatch the essences pertaining to life to the place where they are supposed to go. There is a foundation, something reliable in life that is built for life. I am a living being, and because I am a man and not a pig or a hawk or whatever, there are things that come to me and they will make this self that I am through a process and a motivating factor which is the essences. So there is a connection between living, coming and being and the status of essences.

line 15: *liang jing xiang bo wei zhi shen*

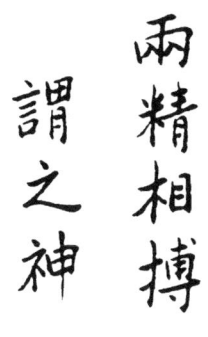

謂之神　精相搏

Then the character *jing* (精), essences, is taken again with *liang* (兩) which means a couple. A couple of essences. This implies that they are embracing each other. The essences coming from one part, and essences coming from another part joining together, they make a couple of essences. And through this mutual exchange something arises, and this is called *shen* (神). Does that mean that one essence plus another essence does not make essences? Yes, they are still making essences, they are making a couple, they are not disappearing, but they are producing an offspring from that meeting, and the offspring is spirits. So it means that the spirits come of their own accord whenever essences are joining together.

Elisabeth Rochat: In these first three propositions we have seen the arrival of life at the universal level, and this life is a junction. We must have the virtue, the *qi*, heaven and earth, and this exchange, this compenetration is what we call life. Or it is called the 10,000 beings, which means everything that is alive. Chinese thinking is not so abstract. In French or in English it seems to be very abstract, but in Chinese it is quite real. It is a very concrete image.

In line 14 this is taken up again:

gu sheng zhi lai wei zhi jing
故 生 之 來 謂 之 精

When there is something living that has arrived, life, greenery on the trees, the tides and the seasons, all that comes and goes: when spring arrives it means that there was something that made spring. And the same for autumn and all the other seasons. So when there is a living being, there must have been something to make it, and that is the essences, *jing* (精). The essences themselves are a junction or a composition, if not they could not make the sub-stratum of life, since life, as we saw here in the first three lines, is itself a junction. So this living being arrives, *lai* (來), and it is there because it has a primordial composition or compenetration which makes its own individuality or specificity, with its own species, that is to say a human being and not a tree or an animal. Each one is an individual within the whole species, and it is the *jing*, the essences, that ensure that I remain myself and you remain yourself. The first line refers to the specificity, the individuality, of each being, and the second line moves on to reproduction, and ends with the production of *shen* which is the 'becoming' of a new being. We will follow that in the succeeding sentences.

Claude Larre: I feel that something has been lost in the translation and it has something to do with the use of the word 'becoming'. It is not enough to have this model or frame to ensure the preservation of the identity of the self, that I remain myself and so on. More than this, the Chinese felt that we need something else to lead life, because it is not quite enough just to be oneself.

48 • THE HEART IN LING SHU 8

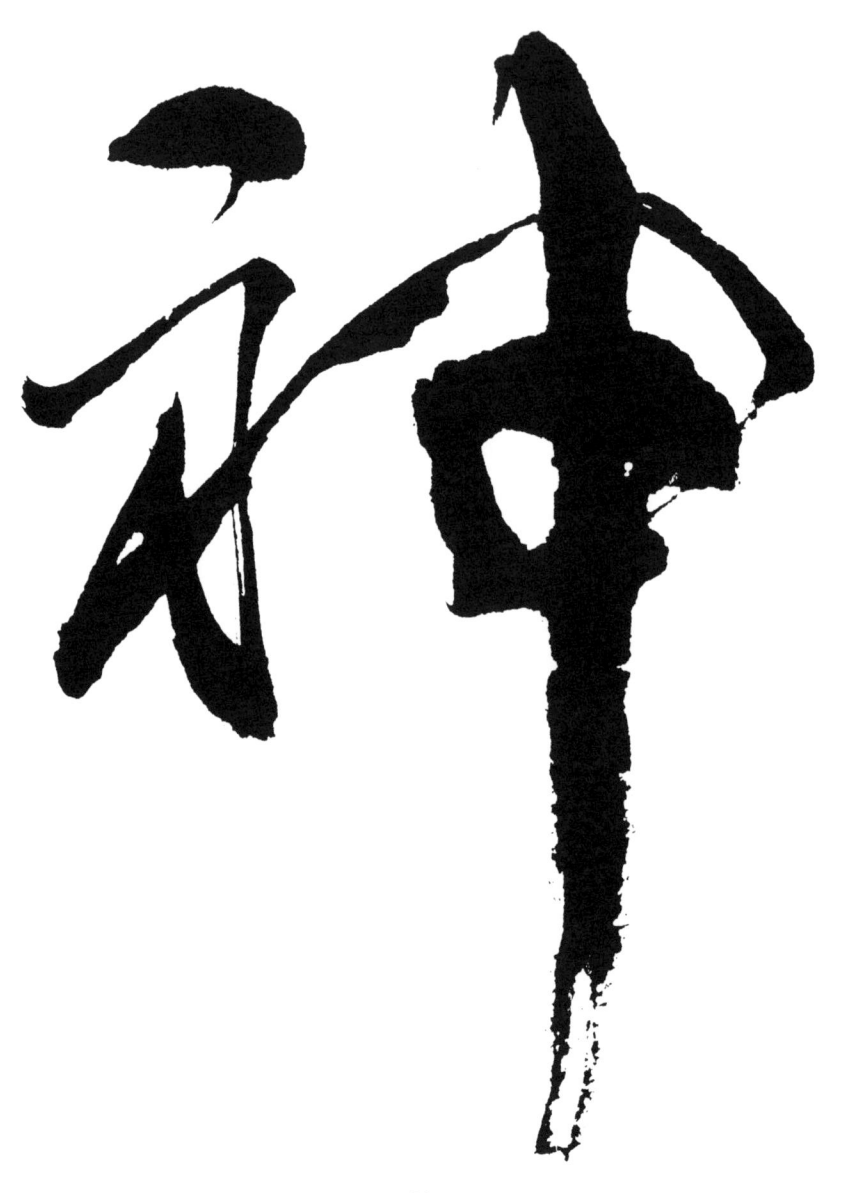

shen 神 spirits

We exist in a way that develops. We have a future. As long as we are living, we are living for something, we are living for tomorrow, and for the years to come. However long, life is not without prospect. Is there any power to take care of the 'becoming'? Yes, there are leaders within us, and we call them spirits. The true role or function of the spirits is not to give us the high mark of spiritual life in general, it is to give us specific guidance for every moment, for every circumstance of our present daily life. Am I strong enough to do without those essences from heaven, to do what is requested, not only to preserve myself with the identity of the essences, but to move my life accordingly under any sort of circumstances? I am not strong enough to do that by myself, or if you prefer, my self has to be taken altogether with a lot of heavenly essences - these are the spirits, and the spirits are riding on myself, as if I am the horse and they are the cavalry men. That is the Chinese concept. It is the essences plus the *shen*, that which is at the same time identity and future.

Elisabeth Rochat: The essences do not exist in the form of some kind of living tissue from which each person draws their substance, because life always has to repeat itself according to the same model, and that is this pattern of the junction or joining together of heaven and earth. It is for this reason that two essences have joined together to produce the new being which is characterised by *shen*. These two essences can be taken at any level that you wish. It is of course the essences of the man and woman who are going to have a child, and on a larger scale it can be the *yin* and *yang*, fire and water, and all that combines together, not only to allow life to appear, but also to provide a dwelling place for the spirits.

Claude Larre: It is quite usual in the Chinese text to have a double meaning. They always tend to use two characters, and in the crossing of the characters something new appears. The difficulty in trying to explain the Chinese text is that when you are discussing two characters you are obliged to give more and more explanation of just one sentence in order to give the feeling that it is not the English text that is being taught, but that through the English language, the Chinese movement of the characters themselves is shown.

Elisabeth Rochat: The essences are a combination, and they can be combined with each other to give another combination which is the essences that are proper to a being, later on these are called the pre-heavenly essences, or pre-heavenly *jing*. Once there is pre-heavenly *jing* then there is something able to attract the spirits, just as if you were to make a little bird house, and then the birds would be able to come inside. This text shows us the conditions of life that have to be prepared in order for the spirits to come, and when the spirits have come then you can discuss all the most subtle forces in man. So then the *hun* (魂) and the *po* (魄) come into the text .

Claude Larre: Elisabeth has been alluding to somebody preparing a nest for birds. But conversely we may prepare birds for nests. There are essences and spirits. What I want to express is the way in which the spirits are coming and the way in which the place is prepared. Also how the essences are disposed one toward the other, and how the essences are renewed through the fact that the spirits are acting.

Elisabeth Rochat: In this text we are shown how the spirits appear. In other texts it is more a question of how the essences proper to a human being appear, and in those texts the *shen* and the *jing* are inverted, so it may say that when two spirits join together that makes the essences which will combine to make a new being. When two spirits join together then that gives birth to a new being, gives form to a new being. Here we are saying that the two *jing* combine to form the *shen.*

Question: Do you mean spirits in a different sense? Are we talking about the same *shen?*

Elisabeth Rochat: Yes, they are the same. What preside over the conception of a new being are the essences and spirits of the parents. Afterwards one splits the hairs, pulls out the threads, for example the liquids of the body, the threads of the spirituality of the person, but it only makes sense if you put them all back together. We are looking at the thread of the spirit, *shen* (神), of the person. We should always look at the text as a thread that we are pulling out and examining, which enables us to see a colour, or to understand something. As the text says, we must always keep the whole in mind.

This is an instinctive and necessary movement, and each acupuncturist should have this feeling at the moment he or she is going to needle somebody. In order to make a diagnosis we look at the different threads and then decide what to do. You can justify everything in it and on the other hand you can justify nothing!

Claude Larre: We have more and more terms but these terms are more and more precise. We can understand the difference between *hun* (魂) and *po* (魄) more easily than we can understand the difference between heaven and earth. We may think that heaven is very clear and earth is equally clear, but that is not true because when we are talking of heaven we are thinking of sky and when we are talking of earth we are thinking of ground. It is just an appearance. Heaven and earth are the most mysterious terms even within our own reality. But when we come to *hun* and *po*, since we know that there are seven *po* and three *hun* and so on, we understand that the text is making more observations. And when we come to the repetition of the verbs *chu* (出) and *ru* (入), to come forth, and to come back and penetrate, it is these movements which are impressing on our minds more than just the expression heaven/earth. Earth is too big to understand. Just consider the mystery of the junction of heaven and earth. Here we are making an analysis which is more a description of the ways life is coming and going, spreading and entering.

Question: I understand the general movement, but I do not understand the position of *shen*. It began with *shen, qi* and *jing,* with *shen* leading.

Claude Larre: We know that the *shen* are the messengers of heaven. The *shen* are always presented as messengers of heaven, and since we have been talking of heaven it is accepted that we are now talking of heaven under another name, and that name is the messengers of heaven. Heaven is not able to be within me without some sort of intermediary, and the intermediary between me and heaven is the *shen.* If we are respecting the *shen* it is because we are respecting heaven. And if we pay attention to the *gui* (鬼), the earth spirits, it is because we have to pay attention to the earth's condition of life.

Each new character is given under the parenthesis of the former. If we are speaking of *shen* we have to speak of heaven, if we are speaking of *jing,* we have to relate that to earth. When we are speaking we have to be like a musician playing, and make sure that we strike the same note at the same time. It might be that there is some difference in timing and then someone may feel that the essences are related to heaven, and another may feel that the essences are related to earth. That is quite normal. It is impossible not to mix the issues if we are not working within the same frame - just as if we were playing music together and we did not start at the same time. And if there is not the appropriate combination of instruments then the music will not be in harmony.

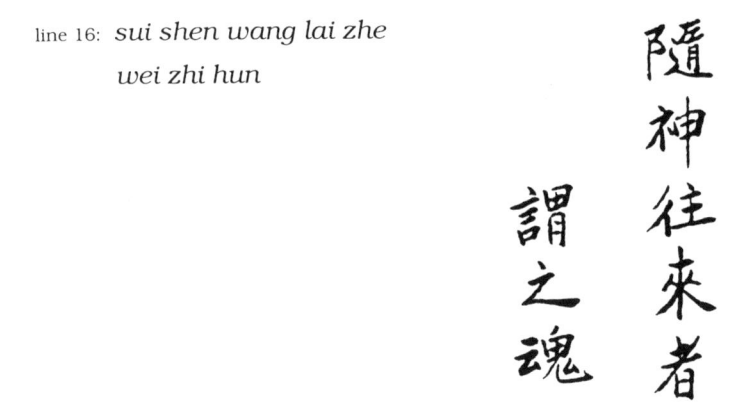

line 16: *sui shen wang lai zhe*
         wei zhi hun

隨神往來者
謂之魂

We are proceeding as in the former two sentences. We want to understand why and how this character *hun* (魂) appears. Assuming that we know what *shen* is we want to understand the *hun* that is dependant on the *shen*. What is the relation between what we call *hun* and *shen*? It is the same thing and it is different. It depends how you are looking at it. And we can see this difference by looking at the way they move.

THE MINISTER'S REPLY • 55

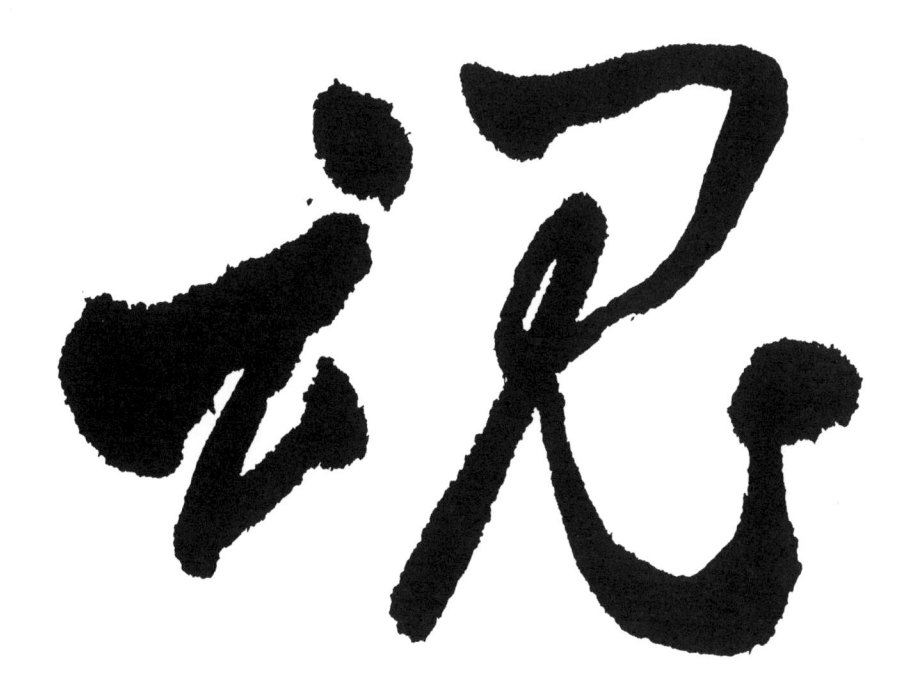

hun 魂

The *shen* are free to come and go, to come into me or to leave and fly away. The *hun* are more like a shadow depending on an object moving under light. They are a sort of escort. The *shen* tend to go up, they want to go back to heaven, and then, within me, a part of my vitality which is called *hun* is on the verge of leaving my body. My family will try to call back my *hun* so that I will not die. As for me, if I want to save my life then I will call back my *hun* myself. And if I am lacking energy because I am too weak, or I have been ill for too long then I will have no more strength, no voice strong enough to call back the *hun*. Then I will die.

Wang (往) is to go outside, *lai* (來) as we saw, is to come back. These two ways of movement, *wang lai*, are the movements needed to create the *hun* from the *shen*. Is it possible to make *hun* from *shen*? It depends how you understand the words. There is no material substance. *Shen* are not some sort of material that you could transform to make *hun*, that is not possible. But psychologically speaking, if you understand that the connection with heaven is made through the *shen*, you may also understand that your most inner self which is less heaven and more yourself, is that face of the *shen* turned towards your own being.

One could say *shen zai wo zhe hun* (神在我者魂), which means that these spirits in myself are *hun*, but the text is not saying that. It was possible to say that heaven in me is virtue. This 'in me' is the largest phrase that we may use to connect 'myself' and heaven. So this connection being understood, we now have to understand what movement the *shen* are making within ourselves, and they are making the motion of the *hun*.

The function of imagination, especially when we are dreaming, by day or by night, is the movement induced by the fact that the *shen* are going out or coming in. They are like the master, and the *hun* are just the companion to that movement.

Question: In pathology, when a patient has attempted suicide, or thinks a lot about suicide, would you, in terms of the spirit, relate that to a loss of the animated self, this *hun*, or would you relate that to weakness in the *po*, like actual survival?

Claude Larre: There are people who are very strong who commit suicide, take the Japanese during the last war. You cannot say it was because the *po* were too weak. But in society in the big cities when people are distressed, they think they want to go to heaven quickly. They are not able to sustain the pressure of their daily life and then this might be a question of *po*. It is never one against the other since life is a mixture, it is a joining of *hun* and *po*, but maybe the prevailing factor in this case is the determination of the will.

In another case it might be a weakness of the kidneys or I

58 • THE HEART IN LING SHU 8

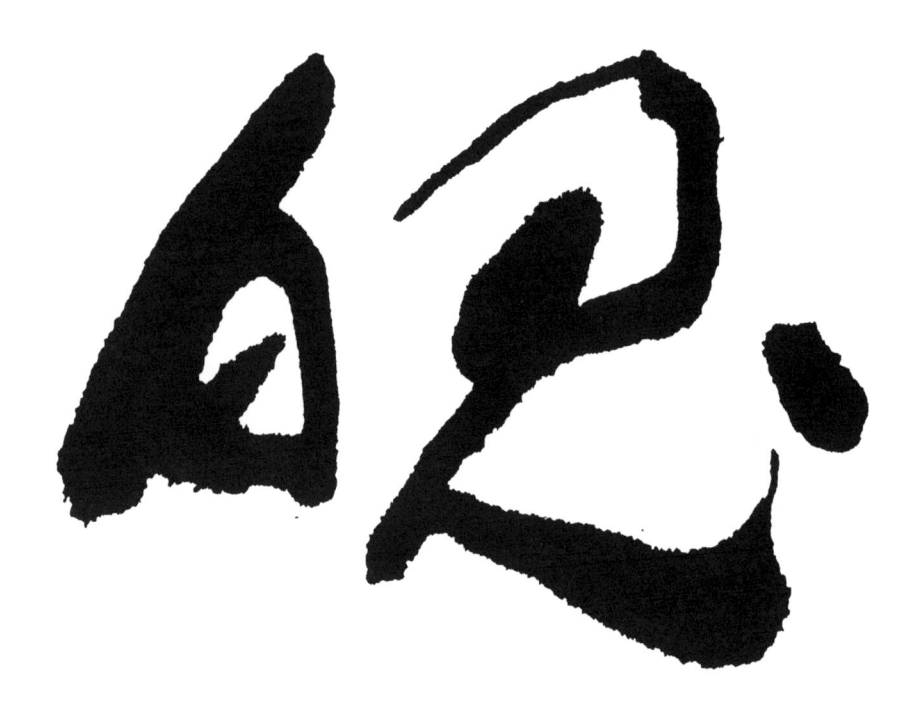

po 魄

do not know what. Then if you restore the fire in the kidneys and the individual is no longer thinking or talking of suicide, then you have the proof that you were right. But if you are treating the *po* and it goes on, then this person has trouble in their mind, the *hun* are not quiet, and then they commit suicide. So why not treat both? It might be safer!

line 17: *bing jing er chu ru zhe*
　　　　　wei zhi po

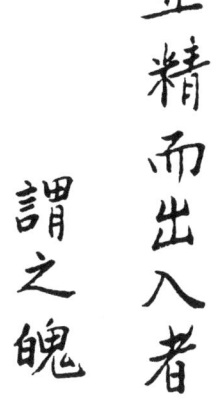

並精而出入者

謂之魄

Hun and *po* are the two sides of life in an individual, so let us try to understand this *po* (魄) character which is contrasted with the *hun* (魂). Now here we have *chu* (出), to go out, and *ru* (入), to penetrate. *Wang* (往) was also to go out but not with the same meaning as *chu*. In *chu* there is the implication of doors. If we are passing through a door or a barrier, then that will be called *chu*. *Ru* is to come back through the door. In both cases there is something to pass through. So this coming and going is more related to earth where there are obstacles. *Wang* is more on the side of heaven where there are no obstacles. The *shen* go and come back as they please, but the *po* go if the door is open, and they come back if the door is not closed - although they may have to knock on the door. The condition of the *po* is not as high as the condition of the *hun*.

In line 16 we saw that *sui* (隨) is to go along, one following the other; *bing* (並) is a different kind of close association. Of course it is a way to go along too, but not to follow, there is nothing to follow here. I will let Elisabeth try to give you more the feeling of the difference between the ways the *hun* are following the *shen*, and the ways the *po* are accompanying the *jing*. You saw already there is a difference here in *chu ru* (出 入), which is not the same as *wang lai* (往 來), and we can look for a similar difference between *sui* (隨) and *bing* (並).

Elisabeth Rochat: The spirits come from heaven and they are the virtue of heaven within us. If you look at the characters for the *hun* (魂) and the *po* (魄) you see that they have one part in common. It is the character *gui* (鬼) which means spirits of the earth, as contrasted with the *shen* (神) which are the spirits of heaven. In *hun* and *po* there is a duality, because what passes through earth comes in the form of *yin* and *yang*. And in the highest aspect of the vitality, when it passes through this taking into form which is the mark of earth, then this spiritual vitality comes out again as a *yin yang* couple, where *hun* is on the *yang* side and *po* on the *yin*. This is discussed in the ancient philosophical texts.

So the *hun* and the *po* are the *yin* and *yang* aspects of the *shen* which are passed into form, and it is easier to grasp them and more possible to define them. We could say that the spirits are present when everything is well ordered. They manifest themselves through the means of expression within the individual which are either of a good quality or not; from that either you radiate and shine or you go out! Within this general picture we can define things more precisely. Firstly we can see within the *hun* an aspect of movement that can reach a long way, for example, imagination, thought, thinking, the mind. You can go a million miles a second with your imagination.

Claude Larre: If you are thinking of something real - I am thinking now of my house in Paris, this is not imagination, this is a recollection of mine. But if I am thinking that I would like to go to a nice place for Easter time, and I know what sort of place - I may think of coconut trees and all that, and I may dream - that is not a recollection, it is imagination, although probably built on a lot of recollections, but they are not real. The important point here is to compare the movement of the will, the movement of the intention and the movement of the imagination, which really go fast and far, and contrast this flying mood with something more constrained, more attached to circumstances and going slowly, and that is the *po* condition.

Elisabeth Rochat: We can remember at this moment that the liver has the function of expansion, putting things into movement and sending things a long way, without forgetting at the same time that its deeper nature is *yin*, storing the blood which serves as the dwelling place for the *hun*. The liver's storage of the blood gives the *hun* this ability to be attached so that it does not fly off. Therefore we have the function of the *hun* in dreams and in imagination, in thinking and in meditation, which is also a very spiritual activity. Meditation is not apathy or inertia, it is an activity which is very calm and very subtle. Everything that is acting in the thinking process, including everything that we consider as intellect and intelligence, all of these things will be the domain of the *hun*.

So why do the *hun* follow the *shen?* If all this world of intelligence, imagination and spirituality wants to remain authentic, that is to say in a true alignment with life itself, then it has to conform to the virtue that is in me - and that is the spirits. It must follow their inspiration, just as earth follows all the inspiration of heaven, and it is through earth that all these different forms then appear.

We cannot be certain that with the *shen* alone there could be ideas and thoughts, but with the presence of the *hun*, then there can be ideas and thoughts, dreams and all that.

But in order to conform to the original, true and authentic life, it has to conform to the initiative of the *shen*.

The *po* are on the *yin* side of the spirits, and in Ling shu chapter 8 it is the reference to the essences which brings out this *yin* aspect of the *po*. The *po* take charge of all that is instinctive in life, everything that is in combination, everything that is entering and exiting, everything that is concerned with the permanent building of life, and at that level there is no difference in nature between *po* and *jing*, the essences. For example, there is an expression, 'The sweat of the *po*', which is a loss of fluids because of an opening up of the pores of the skin, and the sweating deprives you of the internal fluids which are the richness of life in the interior. When this liquid is lost, this function of opening and closing does not work. This is a weakness which is linked with the *po*. The *po* can no longer command the instinctive functioning, which includes everything that comes in and everything that goes out; that you are able to eat, digest, eliminate; that you breathe through the mouth and nose as well as all the pores of the skin. And we can see that the lung is the master of all this field, with the large intestine evacuating.

It is because of this that we have these two words, entry and exit, *chu ru* (出 入). *Chu* is exit, and the first exit is arriving in life, or birth, a coming into being, and the last entry, *ru*, is death, where you return to the earth, to what is formless. Between the two all of life takes place through the composition, the re-composition, the joining together of these essences in a spontaneous and natural manner under the authority of what we call the *po,* as long as the mind does not disturb the process.

Just one last remark. If you look at the 14th, 15th, 16th and 17th lines of the text, working from the right, you can see that the Chinese text adds one character in each line, a character which is not strictly necessary to the meaning of the text, but it creates the image of a staircase which you go down step by step. The text has been made in this way so that you can see the progressive stages.

Claude Larre: We can contrast *sui* (隨), one following the other, with *bing* (並), two persons going abreast, side by side, not following each another. The *hun* are moving behind the *shen,* but I would say that the *po* are going with the *jing.*

Earlier the text says: heaven in me is virtue. Does it mean that if I possess any sort of ability to do whatever I may do, that comes from the fact that heaven is present in me? That is absolutely sure. Does this *de* (德) character have another meaning? Yes, the *de* character has been used to mean to get, to obtain. So we may expand or explain the meaning of *de,* as the virtue to obtain. Then we understand why so many people do not speak of *qi* but of energy, since to get something we need energy, and through this energy or power we are able to get more.

It is just the same as if I have money I am always able to get money, but without money how am I able to get money? So virtue in itself would be some sort of follower, maybe a consort of the *dao* (道). *Dao* would be more expressionless and *de* would be the following expression. There is something more tangible in the virtue than in the *dao*. But if I know something about virtue, from what I know I may be able to figure out something about what I do not perceive.

Elisabeth Rochat: There is some sort of relationship between virtue and the spirits. The spirits are governing the heart and there is the heart in the character for virtue. Another thing is that spirits and virtue have common qualities such as radiance and brightness. It is proper to virtue to shine out, to radiate, just as it is the nature of the spirits to be resplendent. This is part of the most ancient Chinese tradition. The first words of the first Confucian book, which is the little book that all school children learn by heart, is a definition of *dao*. Not in the Daoist sense of the term but in the Chinese sense, that is to say, appropriate behaviour. So the definition of this *dao* is to make the virtue in yourself radiate, and naturally in ourselves it should be brilliant. That is looking at it from a social point of view - virtue should lead or direct your own life, and should direct the life of a nation or a people. In the same way the spirits serve to lead our lives and put things in the right direction to lead an authentic life, so that our lives may give joy to the others around us and give them more life. That is the radiance or brilliance either of the spirits or of virtue.

Claude Larre: To come back to my question on how to understand the difference between *sui* (隨) and *bing* (並). Why do they say in this sentence that the *hun* are following the *shen*, and that the *po* are moving in the same rank as the essences? It might be that the spirits being so similar to heaven, have the freedom which is proper to heaven. But as for earth, earth is absolutely subordinate to the heavenly influx. Earth is concerned with morphology, with places, with walls, doors, openings and various kinds of restrictions which are proper to earth, contrasted to the expanding freedom proper to heaven. Then, if part of the vitality within me, which I call *hun,* is so dependent on the spirits which themselves are dependent on heaven, and heaven is not dependent on anything except the *dao* - if there is so much freedom on the side of heaven, then the spirits are just following, they are not restricted.

To follow somebody who is free is to be free - even if you are dependent, you are free. There is no contradiction in the Chinese mind between to depend and to be free. It depends on whom you are depending. But on the contrary, the condition of earth is always to be restricted by the power of heaven in order to give form to what heaven is meant to manifest. Then, for this reason, that part of the vitality which is concerned with building and rebuilding the self - the essences or the motion of the essences which are the *po* - is subordinate to this restriction proper to the earth.

The glory but also the struggle of human kind is that we have to be free on account of our heavenly origin, but to be free we have to restrict ourselves to the earthly condition which is equally our natural condition. So there is no difference between the way things are at the highest level, which is the reunion or compenetration of heaven and earth, or at the level of *yin yang*. There is no difference between the universe and this small part of the universe or small duplication of the universe which is myself. We read in the ancient texts of the state of the authentic man who has completed his earthly tasks and abilities and has become one with the *dao*, he has become a companion to the *dao*, and that is done by strictly following *ming* (命), destiny. Destiny is the mark of heaven in me.

As for the specific verbs or words to describe the *po* (魄) in comparison with the essences, they are *chu ru* (出 入); *chu* being to go out, and the character shows a small plant coming forth from the ground and beginning to sprout, and *ru* being the grain detached from the natural plant, falling down and entering the ground.

So the contrast is between being a companion to what is

most free in the universe, a companion to the *dao*, or being strictly linked with all the contingencies and all the restrictions proper to morphology. Noone can really expand the length of his body or the time of his life, all this is restricted through the species. We cannot live much longer or very much longer than one hundred years, and we cannot grow much taller than two metres. There are certain limits. We have to be content with these two antagonistic situations: that we are as free as we are able to imagine and we are also the most restricted prisoner in life. And the important point is not to mix the issues, not to say, 'I am not free because I am an earthly human', or say 'Since I am free I can do what I want, I do not care for situations as they are - since I am free, I am free'. All that exaggeration is not possible within this context.

It seems that the verbs describing the movement are more important than anything else when the question is what is *hun* and what is *po*. Since we understand that the text comes from the observation of life, it seems that they have decided to describe humanity as *hun* and *po* as far as movement is concerned. This is just one aspect, because another aspect would be that man is *xue qi* (血 氣), blood and *qi*. And we have to accept all these specific terms and the relationships they are making with one another, and the series in which they present themselves. It is impossible to take any two words in that series and see them in isolation. You have to see them in a connecting line and see how they contrast one with the other.

And finally, it would be the reason why for me the character *bing* (並) is contrasted with the character *sui* (隨). There is a leader and there are followers. The leaders are the *shen* and the followers are the *hun* and they are on the side of freedom, which means heaven. The character *bing* is written with a lot of symmetrical strokes, and it is used to represent a carriage drawn by horses where the horses are side by side. *Bing* is used to refer to the *po* and the essences, but here it is not possible to talk of leaders and followers, so instead of leaders I would say models, and instead of followers I would prefer to say all sorts of I do not know what, which are supposed to be conforming to those models. Say it in the best way Tim.

Tim Gordon: Clones!

Claude Larre: That is the way to have the teaching alongside modern physics!

Elisabeth Rochat: Or partners.

Claude Larre: Whenever earth is alluded to, it suggests the horizontal aspect; it is in the spreading outwards that the situation is seen. And when the statement is made in some sort of verticality, there is following, a leader and all that. But partner is a good word, partner is very similar to follower as to the meaning, but the aspect is different.

Question: I wonder if partner is the correct word because the concept of *shen* and the heart implies a hierarchy. It is the other spirits *hun* and *po*, which are part of *shen* ultimately. It is the spirits who come down from heaven into man and find their expression in the complexion and the eyes. We do not have that with *hun*, there is no mention that the *hun* is found anywhere as a physical symptom, but when you have a *shen* problem the *hun* or *po* or will or whatever will also be imbalanced. But the *shen* is monarch fire and the other *zang* are the officials which have to serve them to complete the whole, so there is a hierarchy. Partners as a word makes something equal.

Elisabeth Rochat: The point is that the *po* are partners with the essences. In the text of Ling shu chapter 8 the *hun* are the followers of the spirits, the *po* are the partners of the essences, not of the spirits but of the essences.

The *hun* are specific to mankind. After death the *hun* reach heaven and they survive for a certain time. And this survival depends on essentially two things: on the way you have lived your life, and on the quality of life you have received from your ancestors. It depends on your ancestors whether you are strong enough to survive. The other thing is the cult of the ancestors, the way in which your descendants nourish your *hun* through the cult after your death.

The notion of immortality is not the same in China as it is in Europe. It is not that you have a soul which survives after death and are therefore immortal, the *hun* have a variable time of survival after death. The *po* also have a possible time of survival but here it is the opposite. The goal is that the *hun* should survive for the longest possible time and that the *po* should survive for the shortest.

The desire for life which united the essences and the *po* and which made them grasp each other, must be exhausted at the moment of death in order for there to be dissolution without any regret. But if instead of dying naturally, you perish, for example in a violent or premature death which is rejected by the being, the desire for life remains and continues after death as a kind of greed. This greed will manifest itself as a desire to grasp life in all the other beings around which risk becoming food for this unsatisfied part, and this gives rise to hungry ghosts and evil or dangerous phantoms. And what does it mean to be evil? Just that they are evil for those with whom they come in contact.

Claude Larre: It would be difficult to live with your window overlooking a cemetery. Is it psychological, or is it the fact that there really is something that may hinder your own life? Some people want to have a house that is well disposed for life and the Chinese pay great attention to geomancy just in order to secure more proper ways of life.

Question: So when the *po* are not at rest when someone

dies you get earthly spirits?

Elisabeth Rochat: When the *po* do not dissolve properly, then this power which in a living being is rapacious - the desire to live and eat - that would be called *gui* (鬼) after death, not *po*.

At the beginning of the text we saw the first appearance of life, a specific life which came into being and which then had the possibility of creating another life through the essences and spirits, the *jing shen*. We saw how this creates *yin yang* movement, which at the spiritual level is expressed by the *hun* and *po*. Looking at the text it is possible to see that in the first seven lines these ideas are taken again and again through the characters. But once we arrive at the *po* there is a break in both the construction and the vocabulary that is quite clearly seen in the Chinese text.

Now there is the appearance of the heart. With the *jing*, the *shen*, the *hun* and the *po* we have the whole realm that constitutes the individual human life. The *hun*, the *po* and the *shen* survive the death of the individual. They are more than the construction the individual makes of their life. No one can exist without the *shen*, the *hun* and the *po*, but each individual human life must have a centre and a director who is exactly appropriate to that life. This is the place of the heart. Not the heart taken as one of the *zang* (臟), but the heart taken as the sovereign, the master, and that is what is said in the next sentence, line 18.

line 18: *suo yi ren wu zhe
wei zhi xin*

所以任物者
謂之心

Therefore, when there is something or someone who is capable of taking responsibility or charge of a being, then you can say that there is a heart.

This character for taking charge or taking responsibility for is *ren* (任), the same as in *ren mai* (任 脈). It is to have or be capable of assuming a charge or a responsibility which is vital for life, and that can be the capacity to take responsibility for your own life, or for another life - to take the burden of another life. Here, what we call the heart in an individual suggests that there is a principal, capable of taking on responsibility for all the other aspects of the being. Unity is maintained. There is a place or a void where spirits can be held. There is a centre of reception where the influences can come and go and then be diffused throughout the whole being. There is a capable central government which has the necessary capacity for this charge or duty. And as soon as there is a heart, then we are able to have all the profound, deep movements of the being which are able to

74 • THE HEART IN LING SHU 8

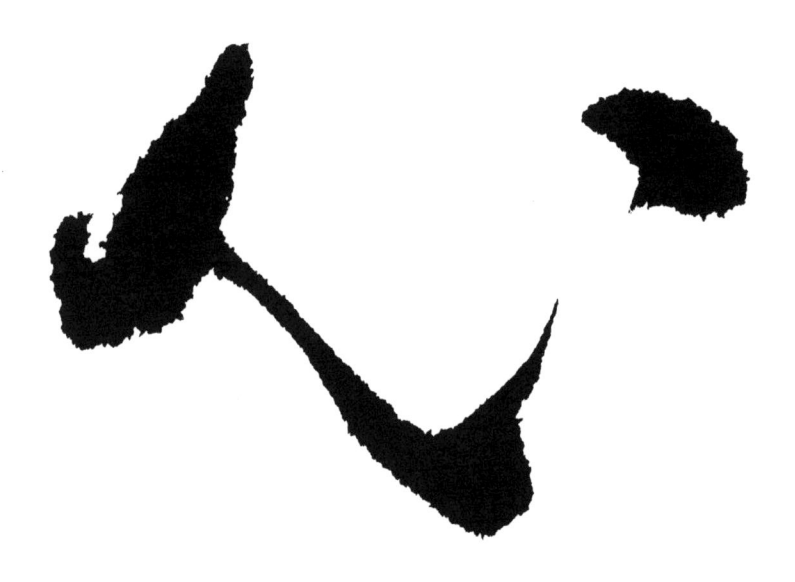

xin 心 heart

guide your life and are as much in the realm of the mind or psyche as in the physical.

line 19: *xin you suo yi*
　　　　 wei zhi yi

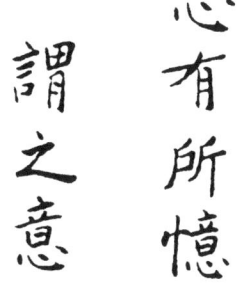

心有所憶
謂之意

Here you can see the same construction of the text where the last character of line 18, *xin* (心), the heart, is taken as the first in the next sentence, creating a chaining or repeating series of these characters. This sentence means that when an idea or thought is presented to the heart, and when the heart accepts it and it does not feel completely strange to the heart, then you can say there is intention, *yi* (意).

The character *yi* (意) is made up of the heart in the lower part, and in the upper part the idea of a sound, or of a note that resounds, like a musical note. It has the meaning of a purpose or intention which has a resonance with the heart - and obviously a note has to be right, a resonance has to be harmonious, it has to harmonise with everything

THE HEART IN LING SHU 8

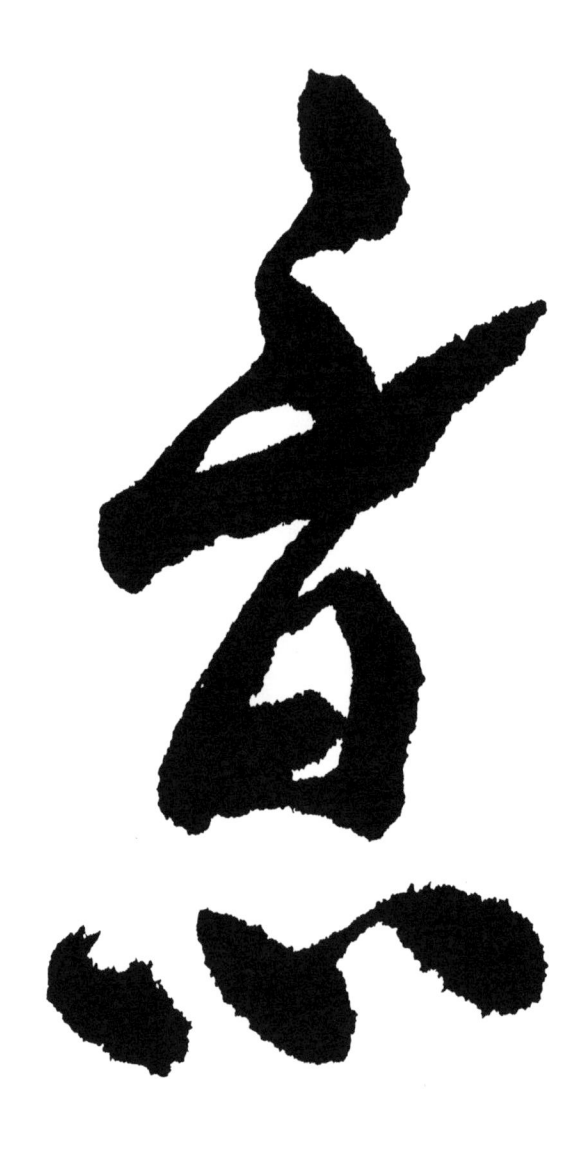

yi 意 intent

that you are deep inside your own being. When you have that right resonance, when it is in tune and strikes the right note, then you have this intent. It is not yet thought, reflection or meditation, it is just the ability of the representation of something to be in tune and in accord with everything that is in you - centralised, harmonised and unified by the heart and in the heart.

line 20: *yi zhi suo cun*
   wei zhi zhi

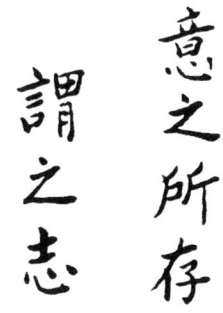

意之所存
謂之志

When this resonance or intention stays, and if it lasts, then you have what is called will.

In the character for will, *zhi* (志), you can see the heart again in the lower part, and in fact the heart is present in all these characters which are the last in each line. So from the moment that the heart appears everything that flows out from it has the stamp of the heart, and this is seen from the characters themselves. The character for the

78 • THE HEART IN LING SHU 8

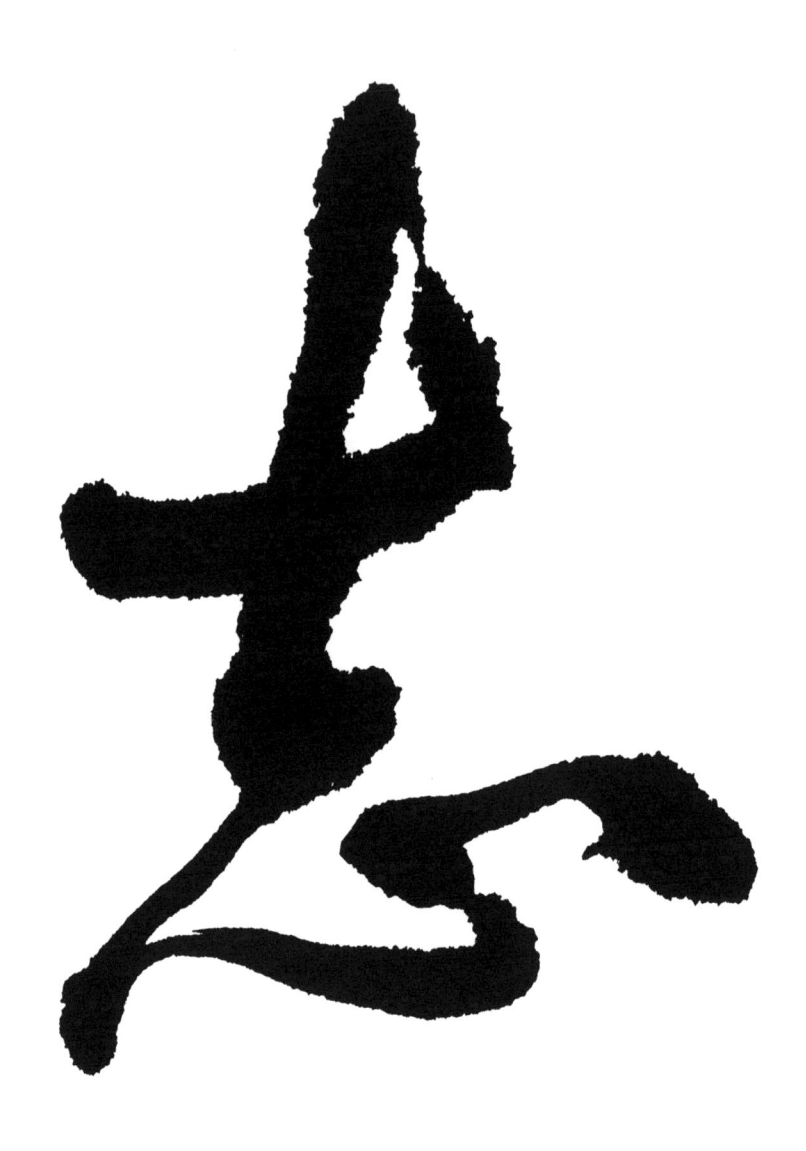

zhi 志 will

will is made with the heart below and the upper part gives the idea of something very virile, maybe the image of a phallus - something that stands up very straight, very firmly, giving the idea of the power behind it. Combined with the heart this gives us the character for will, which is a bit different from what we call will-power in Europe.

Question: Father Larre has said there is a difference between will and wanting. Could you say something about this?

Claude Larre: I would suspect that the wanting implies desire, *yü* (欲). The way is easier when the desire is controlled. Everybody wants everything, that is the Chinese stance. And since there is not enough for everybody then there are struggles for position. We know that. But if I understand that want or desire is normal, I am less afraid of it, and not being afraid of my desires, if I satisfy them at a certain level, I may control them.

If in a room or a house a family is controlling their desires in order to make enough space for talking, resting, studying, for everybody in the family, then most probably, the desires would diminish, the wants would be less felt, and then the will would be built up. But the safest way is to build up the will by control of wants and desires, not by suppressing them. If you tried to supress them, you would deprive yourself of your own vitality, and you may expect a thunderstorm in the future. So, be careful. But if you indulge all wants and desires, then this is the ruin of the will, and your will will fight against the will of others.

Elisabeth Rochat: The construction of the Chinese text changes again in these next three lines. Even if you do not know any Chinese you can see this clearly in the text (lines 21, 22, 23). Now we can see what has already been defined: the heart, with the intent and the will, and before that the *shen*, the *hun* and the *po*, and you will notice that the *shen*, the *hun* and the *po*, along with the intent, *yi*, and the will, *zhi*, form the ensemble which is called the five spirits, *wu shen* (五 神), which are connected with the five *zang*.

Claude Larre: In the same way that the heart is capable of representing the five *zang*, the *shen* of the heart is capable of representing the *wu shen*, the five *shen*. The *shen* is so high that it has the same capacity as the heart to represent other spiritual essences without using their proper names, just by saying the five *shen*. *Wu shen* is the same as saying the *shen* and the others.

Elisabeth Rochat: These are the usual correspondences and in this chapter we see how they come to be. Here we have life and essences, which are expressed in the human being by the *shen*, the *hun* and the *po;* these form the first ensemble which is beyond the life of man. Then we have the appearance of the heart as the sovereign, just as in Su wen chapter 8, The Secret Treatise of the Spiritual Orchid. The heart has the function of sovereign or master, and it is only after there is the heart that there can be a centred person with the possibility of having spirits and making them stay. By contrast, there is the will and the intent, but they are not at the same level.

You cannot put these five spiritual aspects in the cycle of the five elements - there are different levels here. It is the heart which allows the spirits to rest in peace and which by its void and emptiness and tranquillity allows the intent, yi (意), and the will, zhi (志), to exist, without opposing life. There are people who have intent and will which go against their own nature, and there are many illnesses which are linked to that. This situation is due to a heart which is wrongly disposed.

The heart is the residence of the spirits, and if it is capable of being this dwelling place, it has all the good qualities that are necessary to be the principal and commander of all the other aspects, the mental, emotional and physical realms, and all the vital functions of life. Once the heart is established, and relying on this effect, we can continue to define the movements of the psyche.

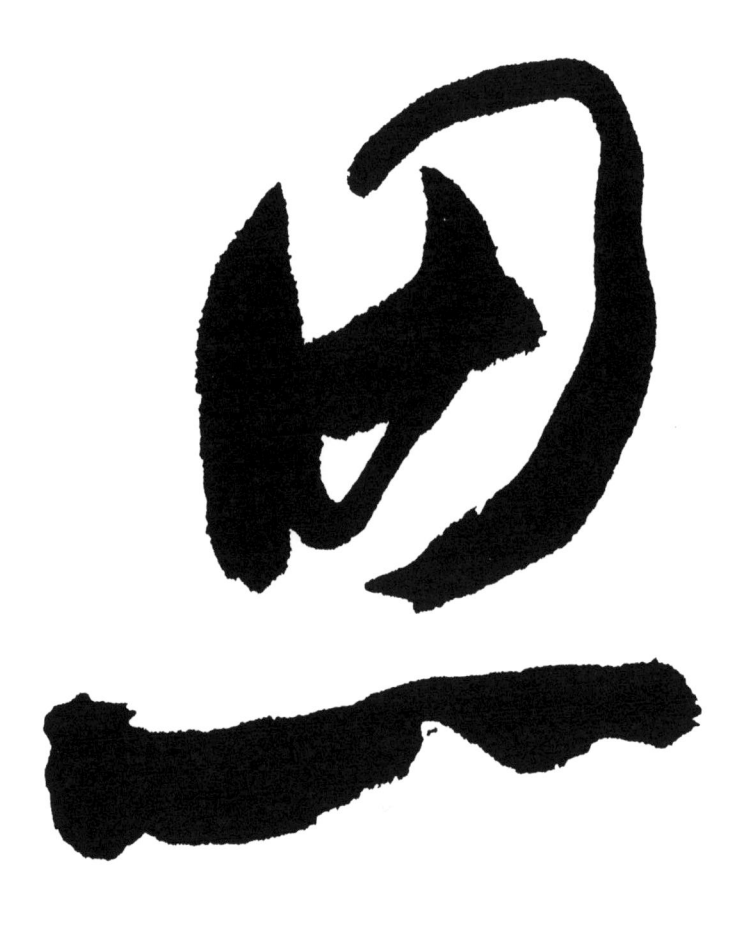

si 思 thought

line 21: *yin zhi er cun bian*
wei zhi si

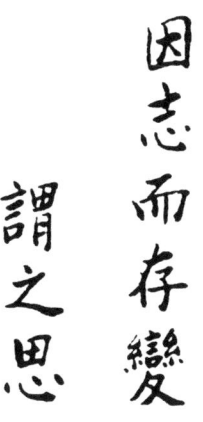

因志而存變

謂之思

The first character in line 21, *yin* (因), gives the impression of relying on an effect, so it is often translated as consequently. The character is the image of a man in prison, he cannot escape; and with all that we have said we cannot escape what is to come. Because of what has been said, this has to follow.

Consequently, the will, when it is there, when it exists, and when it lasts, when it keeps this way of being fixed which is the condition for the will to exist, (you have this idea of duration), and when at the same time it is able to change, then you can say that there is *si* (思), thought.

Here are two contradictory terms: to stay and to change. Here, to change does not mean to change direction like a weather vane. You can stay fixed on something, but also turn and go over the question again and again, looking at all the possibilities of change, and that is what we call thought. There is no hesitation, but it gives the idea of consideration. You look and you mull things over with what you have already considered, and you look at all the movements, all the circumstances which you have already experienced, and through all of that you consider the idea and the will that you have.

In this ideogram thought, *si* (思) you find again, of course, the heart in the lower part (心), and on the top an element which is traditionally explained as being the skull. In the interior of the skull there are some constructions which are thought to represent the brain.

So there is the idea of strict, rigorous construction, and thought, *si*, is the way in which the heart and the brain freely communicate to turn an idea over in the mind, to consider all its aspects and all its possibilities, but the will remains firm and constant. It indicates the direction towards which one is moving, and that does not change. If you do not have this firm direction then it is not called thought. A thought that is not fixed somewhere is just a wandering of the mind.

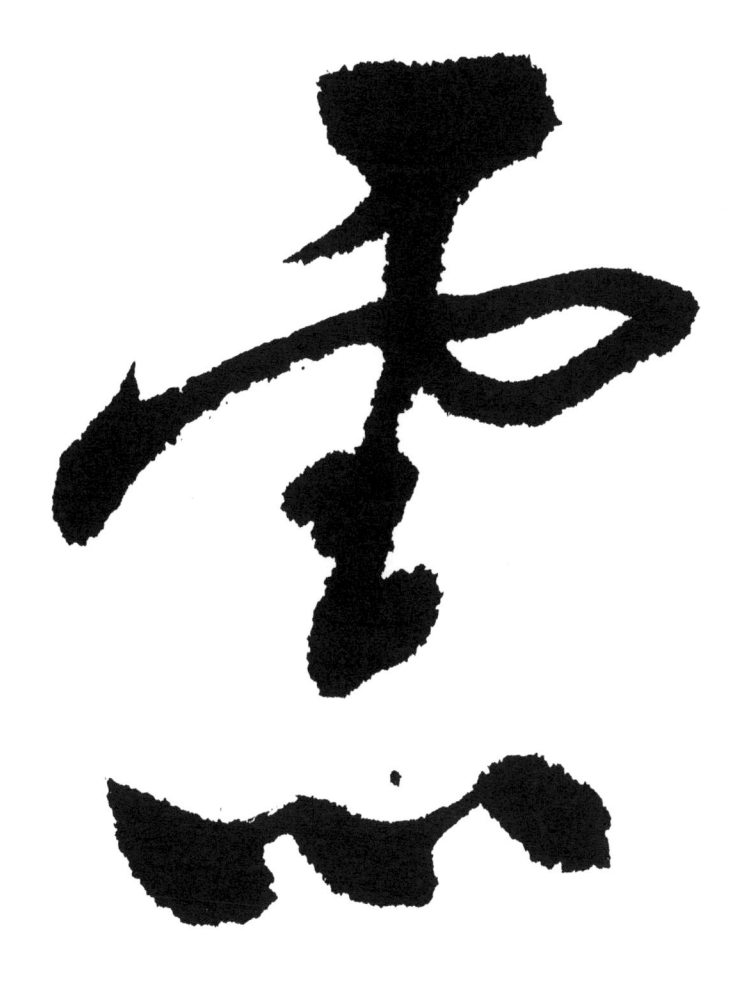

lü 慮 reflection

line 22: *yin si er yuan mu*
  wei zhi lü

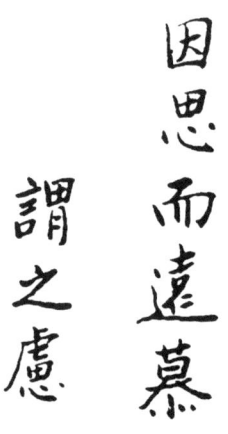

因思而遠慕
謂之慮

When we have a thought, and this thought goes far and goes deep, when it attaches itself to something then a project can be elaborated and can come into being.

There can then be a conception of plans, and this is the same conception of plans that is linked with the liver in Su wen chapter 8. It is not enough that a thought is well constructed and that you turn over all the possibilities, it has, at the same time, to be deeply rooted, so that there is the possibility of it going even further. At that moment there are projects or plans, *lü* (慮), which are made to accomplish something.

Within this character *lü* (慮) we find once again the character for thought, *si* (思). So within the character for planning is the character for thought. In addition there is the character for tiger, or more precisely, the stripes of a tiger. That is to say that all this construction is carried forward - there is projection. This character *lü* does not mean ideas that are formulated any old how. You must not forget that before this there is the heart, the intent, the will and thought, and then we reach the level of *lü* which must be thought of as a plan, a project and also as a profound meditation.

A profound, deep meditation is not just passive, nor is it just a repetition of an old idea, it is the highest aspect of thought.

So, in this character *lü* there are two aspects which only appear to be different when we attempt to translate them into western languages. Sometimes we translate this character as the conception of plans and projects, and sometimes as a contemplative, concentrated meditation. It is the same character; it is a thought which is animated by a movement which pushes it further, and whether that is a project or whether that is a meditation, it has to be anchored in reality, the heart has to be present.

The meditation has to be the source of life, and the project has to be possible or realisable, and it has to be in a good direction for life, so it is a thought that goes a long way, but which has not lost any of its roots. It is always rooted in the heart.

THE HEART IN LING SHU 8

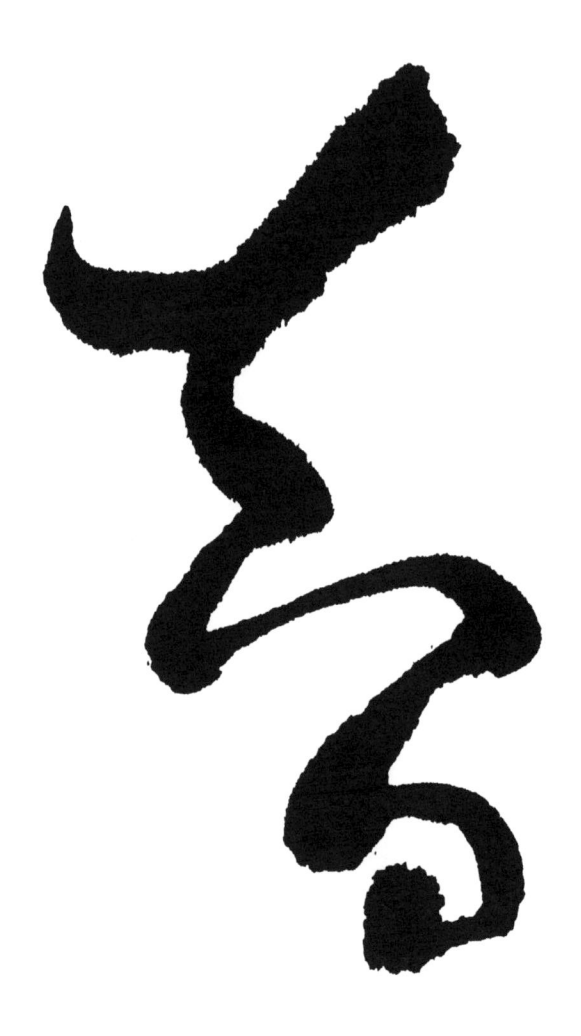

zhi 智 wisdom

line 23: *yin lü er chu wu*
　　　　 wei zhi zhi

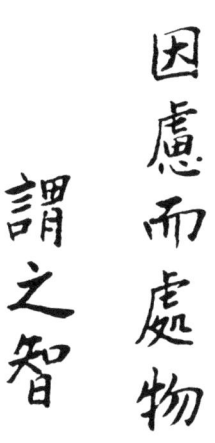

因慮而處物
謂之智

When this meditaton, which is at the same time a project or a plan, can really regulate and administer things, and pass into a phase of actualisation, then you are able to have a practical and active wisdom, which is at the same time know-how or savoir faire.

This knowledge is the upper part of the character *zhi* (知), and when this knowledge is put on top of the character for sun (日), which in this case is also the representation of something coming out of the mouth, then you have a kind of illumination of knowledge, which becomes *zhi* (智), wisdom. But wisdom for the Chinese is always practical. You cannot imagine a distracted sage, or a kind of absent minded professor who has a lot of knowledge in his head but does not know how to do anything. The kind of person who always makes mistakes when he tries to do the simplest practical thing, has a relationship with things and beings which is not correct, and possibly has a weakness in the kidneys, or somewhere else. This would not be a being who is well constructed, he would not have this know-how, this thought in movement to regulate all beings. And this is made clear in the next line:

line 24: *gu zhi zhe zhi
yang sheng ye*

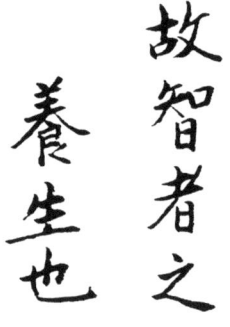

This wisdom is nothing other than to know how to nourish and maintain your life.

'To nourish your life' is made up with two characters, *yang sheng* (養 生). Here we find *sheng* (生), life, which we saw at the beginning, appearing again at the end of this section. The character *yang* (養) gives the idea of nourishing, bringing together all the elements that are necessary for the conservation of life and for growth.

SUMMARY

Elisabeth Rochat: If we look at the whole page of the Chinese text we have first a group of three columns (lines 11, 12, 13) in which life appears in the universe, a coming together of the virtue of heaven and the *qi* of earth in each being and for each being. Then there is a grouping of four columns (lines 14, 15, 16, 17) which show how the spirits of heaven and earth preside over life in each individual.

This presentation, which looks somewhat like a staircase, shows that there is a hierarchy which puts the *shen*, the spirits, in a more honourable place than the *hun* (魂) and the *po* (魄). Then there is a break and in line 18 the heart appears. The heart has to lead life and it leads it in balance and harmony, good proportion and good relationships. You can see that all the terms that are presented at the bottom of each column in this third section have the radical for the heart (心) which marks the supremacy and the presence of the heart in the intimate movements of the being that are represented by the intent, the will, thought and so on. It is not a question of the emotions here. That comes much later on in the text. It is a question of the harmony of all the movements which make life at the highest level.

In the fourth group of columns (lines 21, 22, 23) we have thought, which belongs specifically to mankind. Animals do not retain thoughts. They are distracted, they think of other things. Mankind can retain a thought without obsession, and lead it to a realisation which must adhere to the very current of the individual life. And of course everything presented separately here is a movement that comes together in a human being. But the order of the presentation has to be respected in order to get things correctly formulated.

To use your imagination for plans and projects without anchoring your thought in all of your experience, or without knowing exactly what you want, would mean that you never arrive at the appropriate way of doing something. So the order of presentation that is given here is the natural order for doing things, just as the seasons roll after one another. If not, you are putting the cart before the horse, and putting the cart before the horse indicates that you are leading your spirits against the current.

Now, all the faculties that are mentioned here, the purpose, the will, thought and so on, being governed by the heart, can deviate if the heart is not calm and tranquil, or because the regulation of life is disturbed somewhere. The disturbance could, for example, be from bad diet, or from an emotion that remains too long, or a cold, and that will create an imbalance between all these different movements. Then you may have all kinds of symptoms that appear frequently in Chinese medicine; for example, someone who is always making plans, but who is incapable of taking the smallest decision, or someone who is completely blocked in his way of thinking. This is just to remind you that behind this presentation everything is linked with diagnosis, with symptoms and with treatment. Here we simply have what should be. You cannot act on these spirits, you can just listen to them, and let them govern your life, so that they remain with you.

And from the moment that the heart appears in line 18 we are in a much more precise, a much closer domain, where imbalances appear and can be rectified. Behind this there are the movements proper to the *zang*, and especially the *zang* taken all together and related to the heart, which regulates this good balance. Then you see that all this leads to good conduct and that this conduct comes back to nourishing life, this means that in each thing you follow the natural current which is expressed in the turning of the four seasons: each thing is taken in turn, in the order in which it is presented, making everything turn and revolve regularly.

The beginning of chapter 15 of the Su wen says that it is proper to the spirits to assure this subtlety of permanent revolution, the regular distribution to make everything flow. You have to regulate or balance everything in nature that appears as cold or heat, and that manifests in ourselves as anger or joy etc, either too much activity or inertia. And all this must be balanced through all the cycles that are known in life. It is through this that you can nourish your life.

So this text does nothing but show the natural current of life that is proper to mankind, which is in the spirits and under the government of the heart.

Claude Larre: All that is the answer given by Qi Bo to the question from the Emperor, so we have to see it in the context of the beginning of the chapter. If we consult the text, we see that each of the demands of the Emperor has been answered properly, but we may add one or two remarks on points which are now secure.

The first point in the answer is that heaven and earth are called in. Heaven and earth are the parents of mankind. This is seen in Huainan zi at the beginning of chapter 7 which says that your parents are not your real parents, your real parents are heaven and earth. If we do not stick to that meaning, if heaven and earth are taken as some distant actors in our lives, then we miss the point, and we miss the Chinese perspective on life.

Another point is that life, which here is the character *sheng* (生), (line 13, 6th character) concerns the coming together of heaven and earth to produce life. But this coming together of heaven and earth is more specifically the coming together of *de* (德), the virtue of heaven within me, and the *qi* (氣) of earth within me. We have to keep in mind that I am nobody without the virtue of heaven. It is impossible just to have an ordinary life. Each of us has an extraordinary, perfect, individual and uncommon life. Everything is dependent on the virtue of heaven, and everything is dependent on the *qi* of earth. But we cannot take this as the only formulation of fact in individual life. We can take this as a very well connected line to understand how things are going, to know more about the essences, about the spirits, about the *hun*, the *po*, the knowledge, the know-how, and so on.

A third point is the particular treatment given to the essences. The character for essences, *jing* (精), appears before the actual individual life is given. The text says that the coming of life is through the essences and is marked by the essences. It means that the human species is something that has to be thought of before the actual being is created; and the pre-eminent role of the virtue of heaven is to give the pattern before the making. If there were no pattern, the spirits would have no place to rest, and that is what we were saying previously, that a nest has to be prepared for the birds. Some spirits would come here because the place is convenient for them, and the spirits of man are not being mixed with other spirits which may dwell elsewhere. (Though we have some cases where this is so, for example in Huainan zi chapter 2 we have an individual who at times seems to be a man, at times a tiger.)

So we can understand that in superstition and in all the

creative imagination of the Chinese it is possible that they have the idea of man's spirits mixed with other elusive entities. But the *jing* (精), essences, for human beings, and the *jing* for the clan and for the family is really the model, the fabric, or the way through which life is able to appear. And that is clearly said in line 14, that without this preparation of the essences, life will not appear, and what maintains life is the spirits. It is as if the essences were more logical, or a secondary category of things compared with the spirits.

It is difficult to find an English or French word to explain the connection between the spirits and essences. We find the same difficulty in relation to the *hun* (魂) and *po* (魄). The *hun* and the *po* are closer to me, but just a duplication of the *shen* and the *jing*. If we understand how the *hun* and the *po* are matching one another, then we understand how the *jing* and the *shen* are mutually acting one for the other. It is the same problem but not at the same level.

I can only repeat what Elisabeth said about the position of the heart. Up to line 17 it is just a matching of essences and spirits or *hun* and *po* in an individual without activity in the mind. I feel that the heart is a mirror, and this appears in many texts, where things, events, affairs, are reflected, or it is the place where they are organised, where they are accepted. The heart is a collector. There is no specific word for describing what the heart is, it is only suggested by the position of the characters, one after another.

The heart is more precisely known at the intersection of two lines. I am interested in the way that the presentation is working in our own mind, and that is very important.

It is impossible that what has been said of the *yi* (意), the intent, would be able to be transformed into *zhi* (志), the will, without the character *cun* (存), to stay. The same is true for the *si* (思) and the *lü* (慮), meditation and reflection or effective consideration of the past; and this is a very important point for modern philosophy.

The time will come when there will be philosophers in the western world who will not be able to create a new philosophy without including what the Chinese have said about consciousness, time, space and all that. Many of them pretend to ignore the Chinese work, and they are just repeating the philosophy of Hegel, Kant, Rousseau and others. But the time will come when they will be quoting the Chinese texts, in good or bad translations, because the question of how the embodied human being reacts in face of life, how life and death is accepted, all this has been said in much clearer terms by the Chinese. So the time will come when that will be a part of modern thinking.

QUESTIONS

Question: It was mentioned before that dreams occur because the *hun* (魂) follow the *shen* (神) and the *shen* are free to come and go. I thought that if one dreams it was because the *hun* are not housed, not because the *shen* are free to come and go.

Claude Larre: We saw in the 16th line of the text that it says: following the *shen* coming and going are the *hun*. So it is impossible to make any distinction between the *hun* and the *shen* when they are going out or coming back home, since one is following the other. We have been discussing this question of reflection. If between *shen* and *hun* there is really no more difference than between an object and its reflection, if they go at the same speed, and one is a messenger of heaven and the other your own proper *hun*, if the only distinction is that the *shen* in yourself are called *hun*, then the question of dreaming is a question of how and why the *shen* are going out, and the answer is given in Zhuang zi chapter 2 where it is said that when you are awake it is not possible for the *shen* to go freely wandering around. Your eyes are open and all your senses are alert. You are fixed to all that you see and that makes sure that your imagination and all your actions and movements are under the strict laws operating in the precise world of the awake.

But when you close your external sensory organs, you

immediately close the rigid structure of your mind and then you are free to go everywhere with your *hun*. And your *hun* are received by other *hun*. It is possible for the *hun* to meet like a ladies club when you are dreaming! There are a lot of references to dreams in other books which rely on Zhuang zi chapter 2, because this chapter is so perfect, and probably so old, that it has imposed its own understanding of how we are free to move outside the body with the *hun*. There is the same thing at the end of this chapter about a butterfly being Zhuang zi, or maybe Zhuang zi being a butterfly, connected with the time of sleep and the time of awakening.

Question: You have said that dreams are a very natural phenomenon, but if different dreams have different pathologies, are they not also a pathological phenomenon?

Claude Larre: Everything is pathological in life because there is no perfect human being. It is a deep pathology. There is no normality here among us. But some are really in a sad condition, some seem to be in rather a good condition. How do I know that? Through their faces.

Elisabeth Rochat: We can say several things about this. There are healthy dreams which are a mark of the freedom of the *hun* which is contacting the deep reality of life in sleep, and when nothing comes to disturb this contact. But if someone is slightly disturbed, either in the spleen, the liver, the lung and so on, that can be felt in sleep. In those circumstances, dreams will give an image of this reality even if it is a picture of a certain imbalance. Therefore in the Nei jing there are different diagnostic indications linked with specific organs and the objects about which you dream. It is also possible to have dreams which shake you up and disturb you deeply, and this is an indication of a severe imbalance between the *hun* and what should stabilize the *hun* in the interior. For example, it may be linked with an insufficiency of the *yin* or blood of the liver. You must not forget that the blood carries the spirits to the heart and the liver, and that the liver stores the blood, especially in sleep and at rest. The blood that is not used in the efforts and actions of waking life returns to the liver. And here we find the joining of *yin* and *yang*, of blood and spirits and the *hun* participating in the balance of the being during sleep.

Also in sleep the *wei qi* (衛 氣), the defensive *qi*, which is no longer active on the outside of the body, comes back inside the organs with a two-fold effect: the closing of all the orifices and even of the pores of the skin, and the action of regulating the actions of all the organs at a very deep level, which is the function of the *wei qi* during rest. Rest in a well regulated life should always correspond with the concept of night. This is the ideal proposition.

Claude Larre: Dreams are possible when we are awake, but they are not called dreams, they are called day-dreams. A day-dream is possible since you can be operating with only your eyes and your ears, but other parts of your senses are not alert. So being disconnected with the intense application to the surroundings, you are not free to go everywhere as in true dreaming, but you are freer than now. Some are really day-dreaming now, but others are trying to understand what we say! They are hearing and they are looking, and for that reason it is not easy for them to dream peacefully. Those who are strong enough and brave enough to be day-dreamers, those are half-way between what is needed to do something and what is needed to be done. Because when you are in a dream, you are more done to than doing. But if you are done to in a certain manner, then it proves that you are surrendering to that sort of eruption in your life. If you are weak in certain parts of your body or life, it will be through that weakness that this sort of dream will be acting.

I remember myself, during the month of December I was rather tired and I was unable to fix my mind on listening to people, and I was able to teach without really knowing what I was teaching, I had just a very vague control over what was flowing from my mouth, which is perfect. People like that - but they feel constantly concerned, because they themselves are taken into this way of thinking which is not far from a dream. And we know that we prefer dreaming than facing things to be done. Is that pathology? Yes, definitely. Weakness of the kidneys or the spleen, probably not that of the liver, the liver being overactive in contrast to the weakness of the others. If the condition becomes serious, the heart itself would have a feeling of emptiness, but not a good emptiness, some sort of *xin xu* (心 虛), emptiness through lack of vitality.

Elisabeth Rochat: This is an extract from Su wen chapter 80, which shows the kind of dreams that are connected with the heart:

'When the *qi* of the heart is empty, then you dream of fires and *yang* beings such as dragons.'

And in Ling shu chapter 43:

'When the *qi* of the heart rises up in power then you dream that you laugh easily, or that you are fearful. And when there is a counter-current which allows perverse energy to attack the heart, then you dream that you see hills and mountains with fires, and fires with smoke.'

The first shows the exuberance of the fire of the heart, and the second a deep injury to the kidneys, or a disturbance in the relationship between fire and water.

Question: There has been no mention of the emotions, are we awaiting the subdivision of the *zang* before we mention that?

Elisabeth Rochat: They come later in the chapter where we find all the varieties of emotions which injure life, and then all the symptoms which follow.

Question: But we cannot consider them only as pathology.

Elisabeth Rochat: This is all linked with the void or the emptiness of the heart, the art of the heart. When you name an emotion, when it appears sufficiently strongly to actually take root in your being, that means it is not in balance with all the other movements, and therefore it is pathological. In the balanced harmony of life, in the circulation and movement through the heart, what pushes you upwards must be moderated by what pushes you downwards. What pushes you outwards must be balanced by what goes inwards. At that moment it is like a car that is working well, with no little noises. When you get those little noises, then that indicates that you are sad or angry, it shows that there is disharmony. One movement stays at the expense of all the others. At that moment then you are in anger. But if that movement of anger is well balanced by considerate thinking, by prudence, then there is no more anger, and you move forward.

Claude Larre: When Elisabeth was saying that we balance one of the emotions with the other, I am sure that you understood that this was not to achieve a standstill. It was that for that period of time you will be more powerful, or you will be more grieving, and so on; like the birds singing in the early morning in spring. There is no way to stop them, and there is nothing wrong. It is pathological only when you are unable to stop that emotion, even when you want to.

Elisabeth Rochat: For example, it is normal that rains come from time to time, and that it is windy from time to time. But if it rains all the time, or if it is windy all the time, then we say the weather is crazy. In the Chinese text there are many comparisons between the weather and the emotions in man. They are exactly the same thing.

APPENDIX 1

APPENDIX 1

The following is an extract from a commentary by Claude Larre and Elisabeth Rochat de la Vallée on Nei Ye, chapter 49 of Guan zi. This commentary was given after the presentation of Ling shu chapter 8 and it gives an excellent illustration of the heart from a non-medical text. We are unable to reprint the whole text, but offer a small extract here and urge readers to consult the original text. (The English text referred to here is translated by W. Allyn Rickett, and published by Hong Kong University Press)

THE ART OF THE HEART

'When our hearts are well regulated, our senses are well regulated too. When are hearts are at rest, our sense organs are at rest too. What regulates them is the heart. What sets them at rest is the heart. The heart thereby contains a heart. (That is to say) within the heart there is another heart.'

Elisabeth Rochat: The terms that are used in the Chinese are just this - the heart is to store the heart. In the middle of the heart there is another heart. So the question is whether this heart which is the middle of the heart is the consciousness, intelligence or the mind. I feel this interpretation would reduce the Chinese thinking. If they had wanted to say that within the heart was thought or mind then they would have been forced to use another character. This would be a limitation as the heart is the sum of everything that makes life - intelligence, thought, sensation, emotion, etc. Everything has to circulate and be transformed through the power of the heart, and it is that that makes the quality of life in a human being.

At the same time we can understand what is written in the old medical books, where we have a heart which is protected by a heart. And from time to time they speak of this central heart which is nothing but a void, a possibility of transformation, transmutation and circulation. This void is filled with the spirits which make all this circulation and transformation, and which allow it to stay within my own being and my own unity, so that my life is not the life of another.

We so often undrstand the heart on a more tangible, more visible level, with a particular action, and this is seen in the image of fire. But here it is not the free circulation and flow of everything, but more the specific circulation of the qi and the blood, and it is in this sense that the heart is said to master the mai (脈). It has mastery over the vital circulation which forms the blood. The character which is used to express this mastery is zhu (主), and you can see how this differs from the function of the prince, jun (君),

which was the character used just now in the text. In Su wen chapter 8 the charge of the heart is both of these together, *jun zhu* (君 主) the prince and the master. It is at the same time this void, this emptiness which rules and regulates everything, and the expression of life at the level of the heart and of fire, for example, through all the animating network making blood and *qi* circulate.

So we can see that the French and English translation 'master of the heart' or 'heart governor' is not at all correct. It is not the master of the heart - the heart cannot have a master! The text continues:

'In the heart of that heart, intellect comes before words.'

Here you see that intellect, *yi* (意), (which we have preferred to translate as intent or purpose) exists before things have come into words.

'After intellect come forms, after forms come words, and after words come implementation. After implementation (things) will be well regulated. If they are not well regulated, there will certainly be confusion. If there is confusion, there will certainly be death.'

The character which is translated as 'will be well regulated' (*zhi* 治) is one that is used for governing things well, or to treat a patient well, or to cure a patient - because all of that is the same thing.

'When the essence exists (within) and gives life naturally. The outer appearance will then glow. Being stored internally, it acts as a fountainhead. How great! Being peaceful it acts as a wellspring for the qi of life. So long as the wellspring does not dry up, the four parts of the body then remain firm. So long as the wellspring is not exhausted, the passages of the nine apertures then remain clear. Thus it is possible to explore the limits of heaven and earth and reach all within the four seas. If within there are no doubts, there will be no calamities without. If the heart is complete within, the form will be complete without. Neither encountering the calamities of heaven nor meeting with harm from men. We call such a person a sage.

'When a man is capable of being correct and quiescent, his flesh is full, his ears and eyes sharp and clear, his muscles taut, and his bones sturdy. Thus he is able to wear on his head the great circle (of heaven) and tread on the great square (of earth).'

Here we can see that with a heart which is in harmony and well centred, the man is in his correct position between heaven and earth. This is seen right down to the quality of the pores of his skin. A sage has a clear complexion. That is said everywhere.

'Concentrate your qi until you become spirit-like, and all things are complete (within). Can you concentrate? Can you adhere to the unity of nature?...

...When the four parts of the body have become corrected and the blood and qi have become quiescent, you may make your intellect adhere to the unity of nature and concentrate your heart... It is ever so that the life of a man must depend on impeturbability and correctness. The way in which they are lost is certain to be through joy or anger, sorrow and suffering.

For this reason, to put a stop to anger there is nothing better than poetry. For getting rid of sorrow there is nothing better than music. For moderating music there is nothing better than the rites. For preserving the rites, there is nothing better than respect. For preserving respect there is nothing better than quiescence.'

Claude Larre: It takes time to see the fitness of each of the determinations. Our work, as far as I understand it, is not only to understand, but to look at the text as if it were not possible to say anything differently, and to look at another text and have that same feeling. It has to be said in this way. Then any so-called contradiction is erased by the fact that the modern mind is free to change its point of view. That is typical of the traditional text.

APPENDIX 2

APPENDIX 2

The following is taken from a talk given in November 2002 by Elisabeth Rochat de la Vallée at the Pacific Symposium, San Diego. It draws on non-medical texts to explain the Chinese concepts of the heart, the spirits and the emotions. The talk was edited by Sandra Hill.

To be human is to be self-conscious and self-aware. One consequence of self-consciousness and self-awareness is confusion and fear, and each civilization has addressed this fundamental human problem by developing its own system to facilitate human life and ensure a feeling of security within an often hostile universe. Early animism, ancestral worship, and the various levels of understanding of heaven (tian 天) are part of the attempt by the Chinese to create their own system.

Before the Christian era, the Chinese built a vision of the universe where every phenomenon is related to every other phenomenon as part of a gigantic web of cosmic life. This is generally called the system of correspondences and is widely used in theories of medicine. Independently and correlatively, the theory of qi (氣) was developed. Qi is behind any form, any phenomenon, any manifestation, and determines the quality and characteristics of every form, phenomenon and manifestation. *Qi* is what links together phenomena of analogous qualities or activities; it is potential becoming life, providing the transformations at work in any living being. Everything that occurs at any level within a human being is dependent on *qi*, whether it is physical, physiological, psychological or mental. Health, disease and treatment are all a matter of *qi*.

In nature, *qi* is acting regularly, as if following an order. This natural order is seen everywhere. One of the best and most traditional examples is the four seasons, sometimes referred to as the four *qi*, which represent the alternation as well as the composition of *yin* (陰) and *yang* (陽). *Yin* and *yang* are not exactly two types of *qi*. They are rather the *qi* moving through various phases, according to time and circumstance. Hence the *qi*, expressed as *yin* and *yang*, expands and contracts during the four seasons, provoking various reactions and determining all the aspects and cycles of life. There may appear to be irregularities in the course of the seasons, some particular *qi* or wind may not be in the right place at the right time, but basically the system works and spring inevitably follows winter, as autumn follows summer.

In the few centuries before the Christian era, the evolving notion of *qi* supported the elaboration of the system known as the five elements, agents or phases. This is a way to classify all living beings and phenomena, all kinds of qualities and cycles, and put them into a precise relationship, in order to present their interplay and establish the pattern of their mutual influence, alternation or succession.

So what makes the *qi* act with such regularity? What makes the *qi* of each season change at a particular time? What makes the *qi* appropriate to each of the five elements/phases act according to its own type, wherever and whenever it is appropriate?

From a certain point of view, the spirits (*shen* 神) could be seen as the power of change, making sure that the *qi* is at the right place, and in the appropriate way. For instance, there is a spirit of the water element making sure that the *qi* expressing the mode of activity proper to the water element is working correctly; there is a spirit of the river, making sure that the river flows as it is supposed to and so on. These powers, these spirits, are deities, souls of the dead, and certainly they also become - at least for the scholar - representative of heaven, as heaven is the natural order of life.

'Perceiving the way of change and transformation is how one perceives the spirits.' (Yi jing)

The universe is seen as a self-regulating system, with its regulations in the rhythms and cycles expressed through the theories of *yin* and *yang* and the five elements. This organization is the pattern for any being or phenomena, including the human being. All capacities, activities, movements, transformations, affinities are *qi* regulated through this system.

But it seems that within the human being this movement of *qi* can go wrong. It moves in the wrong direction, it gets blocked, knotted, dissipated, and finally it works against life. And this is not merely the result of a flaw, a defect in the constitution or even due to inescapable circumstances. This disturbance of the *qi* may come from wrong behaviour, bad diet, careless exposure to cold, and even the exhausting use of sensory or intellectual abilities.

So how can human beings act against life in such a way? It is because within the human being there is obviously a tendency for the life giving or life maintaining *qi* to operate against life.

And here we come to the heart (*xin* 心). The heart is the very centre of the human being and the very centre of the self. It is a collection of all perceptions, sensations, information, memories, knowledge, tendencies, ideas, thoughts, desires and emotions. It is the whole of emotional life, but also the mind, the psychology, the intelligence. In Chinese thought, the heart is 'myself', it is 'me'. The heart reacts to any event, situation, circumstance, stimulation. And, as we see in Lao zi chapter 55: 'The heart activates the *qi*.'

It is said that the heart is responsible for the correctness or for any distortion in the course of the *qi*. And that is dependent on the way that the heart (or the way that each individual) is able to follow the natural order or to deviate from it. The natural order is given to each individual at the beginning of life as the 'proper nature'. This proper nature is necessarily part of the great cosmic movement of life, and is in conformity with the maintenance of life.

This does not necessarily mean that there is no flaw in the genetic inheritance - but this would be considered as part of the human transmission, an alteration due to human behaviour through an ancestral lineage possibly going back several generations. Neither does it mean that there will be no disturbance during pregnancy and in the early stages of life, which may effect the way the heart is able to develop. But it does mean that there is always the possibility for each individual to access the natural order of life within themselves. To follow this natural order is the only way not to dissipate or waste vitality.

When the *qi* is operating correctly and harmoniously, then the material matrix, the essences (*jing* 精), are rich and abundant. Because of this, the interplay of *qi* and essences works most efficiently, and all the vital functions work well. This perfect functioning is seen in the presence of the spirits. Thus the term 'vital spirits' is expressed in Chinese by *jing shen* (精 神), essences/spirits.

So what is it that goes wrong with the human heart, with the *qi* and consequently the spirits?

Because the human being is self-conscious, there is this self, this 'I', and the heart reacts with self-consciousness, which gives us not only the ability to perceive, but also the possibility of self-knowledge. Not only do I perceive, but I know that I perceive. I know that I am, and therefore I know that one day I will be no longer. This consciousness, which is what makes us human, also destabilizes a kind of natural functioning, and we are no longer able to act instinctively or unconsciously.

Therefore, in response to stimulation and events, the heart reacts with exaggeration, defensiveness, fear, excitement, and it is human destiny - the task of each human being - to put the heart back in harmony with the natural order. This is our daily practice, to apply ourselves to giving back to the heart this ability to react appropriately, without the need for excitement or exaggeration, fear or blockage.

'By nature, humans possess blood and *qi* and a heart that allows knowledge. Grief as well as joy, elation as well as anger do not exist permanently within. They are reactions to the incitement of external things. It is then that the art of the heart intervenes.' (Liji Yuji)

The reactions of the heart depend on the inner disposition, the tendencies, ideas and emotions which are within the heart. It is common experience that we do not react to the same words coming from someone we like and someone we do not like. If we are full of elation and joy, we will not be affected in the same way as when we are sad, defensive or angry. So it is what is inside the heart, what is in the mind (whether or not we know that it is there) that affects all our reactions.

Tendencies, which may be natural, become desires. Desires are harmless if they are the pure expression of life trying to find what is necessary for its own expression, but are harmful if they become exaggerated - to want too much or with too much intensity.

We cannot be without emotions, but we need to know that emotions, because they are always exaggerated, disturb the innermost aspects of our being - the movements and activities of life as operated by the *qi*. Furthermore, our ability to know, think, even to perceive, is all the activity of the heart. So, if any emotion is held in the heart, not only does it disturb the movement of *qi*, but it also alters our ability to perceive, to know, to judge, to feel and to react appropriately.

If the emotion is violent, it may be obvious to others (and even, eventually, to ourselves) that our mind was disturbed, that we were literally 'out of our mind'. But if a prejudice, a dislike, is built gradually and imperceptibly, the damage is even more serious, because we have lost the ability to know or perceive that we are out of our mind.

The 'art of the heart' is to empty the heart every day. It is to reduce what does not appear to be the natural expression of our lives, to diminish the materialistic and psychological needs; to take inspiration from the natural order experienced in the four seasons, and also in the wisdom of past generations, as experienced for example within the ancient rites and rituals. It is to act in such a way that the inner disposition becomes more and more aligned with the natural order, the thought as well as the behaviour and actions. When the heart is able to take in all that is presented in openness, knowledge is able to become wisdom, the kind of wisdom that is nothing other than to know how to nourish life.

LINGSHU CHAPTER 8
BEN SHEN

First section
Text and translation